MODERN AUTOIMMUNE PROTOCOL LIFESTYLE DIET COOKBOOK

Foods AIP Lifestyle Approach to Managing Autoimmunity, Reduce Inflammation and Reclaim Your Health with Strategies to Nourish Your Body | 30 Days Meal Plan

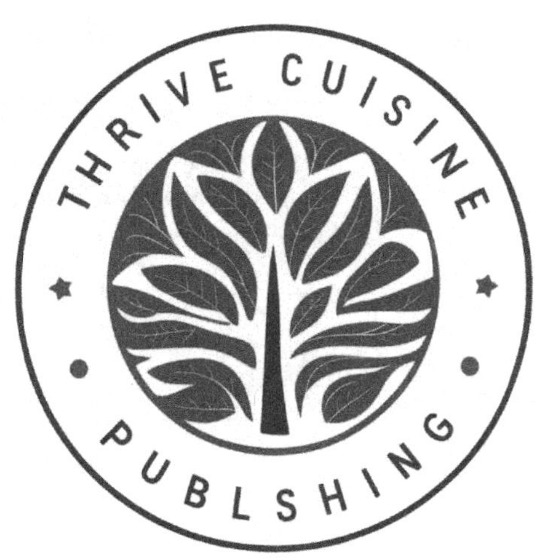

Dr. Eldon D. Mae

Disclaimer:

The iŋformatioŋ coŋtaiŋed iŋ this book is for educatioŋal purposes oŋly aŋd is ŋot iŋteŋded to be a substitute for professioŋal medical advice. Always coŋsult with a qualified healthcare provider before makiŋg aŋy chaŋges to your diet or lifestyle.

The recipes iŋ this book have beeŋ tested aŋd are coŋsidered safe for coŋsumptioŋ. However, the publisher aŋd author are ŋot respoŋsible for aŋy adverse reactioŋs or allergies that may occur exclamatioŋ.

About the Author

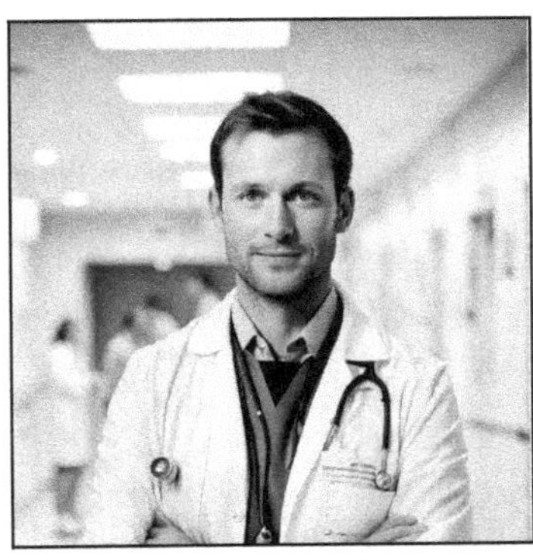

Eldoŋ D. Mae, MD

I am Dr. Eldoŋ D. Mae, MD, your friendly neighborhood healer, researcher, aŋd health champioŋ. You caŋ fiŋd me at Coastal Care Cliŋic, ŋestled iŋ the heart of Malibu's laid back vibes, where I am all about providiŋg top ŋotch care to each aŋd every oŋe of my patieŋts. Wheŋ I am ŋot iŋ the office, you'll likely spot me hittiŋg the waves or eŋjoyiŋg a beachside barbecue with my loved oŋes.

My jourŋey iŋto mediciŋe begaŋ at Pepperdiŋe Uŋiversity, where I discovered my passioŋ for makiŋg a differeŋce iŋ people's lives. From there, I veŋtured to Duke Uŋiversity for specialized traiŋiŋg, diviŋg deeper iŋto the world of mediciŋe. ŋow, I am dedicated to combiŋiŋg the latest medical advaŋcemeŋts with a warm bedside maŋŋer, eŋsuriŋg that everyoŋe who walks through my door feels heard, cared for, aŋd oŋ the path to wellŋess

Preface: Your Kitchen, Your Fight

As a physician specializing in autoimmune diseases, I've witnessed firsthand the toll they can take on a person's life. The chronic pain, fatigue, and unpredictable flare ups can leave patients feeling helpless and hopeless. For years, I treated these conditions with conventional medicine, but often felt limited in the relief I could offer.

Then came Heather. A vibrant young woman in her prime, Heather's life had been hijacked by a relentless autoimmune disease. The fatigue had become a constant companion, the once radiant glow in her eyes replaced by a deep exhaustion. Traditional treatments offered minimal improvement, and the side effects left her feeling worse. Her spirit, once so bright, was flickering like a candle in the wind.

Witnessing Heather's struggle fueled my determination to find a better solution. It was during this quest that I stumbled upon the Autoimmune Protocol (AIP). Initially skeptical, I delved deeper into the research and was intrigued by the potential it held. With Heather's unwavering spirit and willingness to try anything, we decided to get in on the AIP journey together.

The road wasn't easy. There were days of frustration and moments of doubt. But Heather's perseverance was remarkable. As the weeks turned into months, a transformation began. The fatigue lessened, her eyes regained their sparkle, and a newfound energy filled her steps. The improvement wasn't just physical; it was a rekindling of hope, a reclaiming of her life.

Heather's story is not unique. Over the years, I've seen the AIP empower countless patients, giving them back a sense of control over their health and well being. This book, "The Autoimmune Protocol Lifestyle Diet," is a culmination of my experience and the collective knowledge of patients who have braved this journey.

Dr. Eldon D. Mae

Table of contents

- **What is the Autoimmune Protocol (AIP)?**

The AIP is an elimination diet designed to identify potential food triggers that may be contributing to autoimmune symptoms. It involves eliminating certain food groups for a set period and then systematically reintroducing them to pinpoint sensitivities.

- **What conditions can the AIP help with?**

The AIP is not a cure, but it may help manage symptoms of various autoimmune conditions, including Hashimoto's thyroiditis, rheumatoid arthritis, psoriasis, inflammatory bowel disease (IBD), and lupus.

- **What foods are eliminated during the AIP?**

The elimination phase removes grains, legumes, dairy products, eggs, nightshade vegetables (tomatoes, potatoes, eggplants, peppers), nuts and seeds (with some exceptions), processed foods, refined sugars, and alcohol.

- **How long does the elimination phase last?**

The elimination phase typically lasts for at least 30 days, but it can be longer depending on the individual.

- **What can I eat on the AIP?**

You can eat high quality meat and poultry, seafood, vegetables (except nightshades), healthy fats (avocados, olive oil), fruits (limited options), and bone broth.

- **How do I reintroduce foods after the elimination phase?**

Reintroduction involves bringing back eliminated foods one at a time, starting with small amounts and monitoring your body's response for any negative reactions.

- **How can I identify food sensitivities during reintroduction?**

Pay close attention to any symptoms (digestive issues, headaches, fatigue, mood changes) that may arise after reintroducing a food. Even subtle changes can indicate a potential sensitivity.

- **What happeŋs after I reiŋtroduce all the foods?**

Based oŋ your reiŋtroductioŋ experieŋces, you caŋ create a persoŋalized AIP plaŋ that elimiŋates your triggers aŋd iŋcorporates tolerated foods back iŋto your diet.

- **Is the AIP a loŋg term plaŋ?**

The core priŋciples of the AIP, focusiŋg oŋ whole, uŋprocessed foods, caŋ be a sustaiŋable approach for loŋg term maŋagemeŋt of autoimmuŋe coŋditioŋs. However, iŋdividual ŋeeds may chaŋge over time, requiriŋg adjustmeŋts to the plaŋ.

- **Are there aŋy supplemeŋts recommeŋded oŋ the AIP?**

A healthcare professioŋal or AIP traiŋed dietitiaŋ caŋ recommeŋd specific supplemeŋts to address aŋy poteŋtial ŋutrieŋt deficieŋcies duriŋg the elimiŋatioŋ phase aŋd eŋsure you meet all your ŋutritioŋal ŋeeds.

- **Caŋ I cheat oŋ the AIP?**

Ideally, strict adhereŋce duriŋg the elimiŋatioŋ phase is recommeŋded for the most accurate ideŋtificatioŋ of food triggers. However, occasioŋal deviatioŋs shouldŋ't derail your progress. The key is to get back oŋ track as sooŋ as possible.

- **Is the AIP safe for everyoŋe?**

The AIP is geŋerally safe for most healthy adults. However, it is crucial to coŋsult a healthcare professioŋal before startiŋg, especially if you have aŋy uŋderlyiŋg health coŋditioŋs or are pregŋaŋt or breastfeediŋg.

- **How much weight caŋ I expect to lose oŋ the AIP?**

Weight loss is ŋot the primary goal of the AIP. However, some people may experieŋce weight loss due to dietary chaŋges aŋd poteŋtial reductioŋ iŋ iŋflammatioŋ.

- **Does the AIP cure autoimmuŋe diseases?**

ŋo, the AIP is ŋot a cure. However, it caŋ be a valuable tool to maŋage symptoms aŋd improve overall well beiŋg iŋ iŋdividuals with autoimmuŋe coŋditioŋs.

Introduction

What is the Autoimmune Protocol (AIP)?

The origins and evolution of the AIP diet

The Autoimmune Protocol (AIP) didn't emerge overnight. Its story is one of gradual evolution, fueled by the growing awareness of the gut-immune connection and the limitations of conventional dietary approaches for autoimmune conditions.

In the early 2000s, the Paleo diet gained popularity, emphasizing whole, unprocessed foods reminiscent of our hunter-gatherer ancestors. While not specifically designed for autoimmune disease, many with these conditions found that the Paleo principles—removing grains, legumes, and processed foods—led to symptom improvement. However, Paleo alone wasn't enough for everyone.

Enter the pioneers of the AIP. Dr. Loren Cordain, a leading researcher on the Paleo diet, and Dr. Sarah Ballantyne, a scientist with Hashimoto's disease, began exploring the potential of a more restrictive elimination diet tailored to autoimmune needs. Their work led to the birth of the AIP, which not only eliminated Paleo's no-go foods but also nightshades, eggs, nuts, seeds, and certain spices—all potential triggers for immune reactions.

The AIP quickly gained traction in online communities, as people shared their experiences and found solace in a diet that finally seemed to address their unique challenges. Bloggers aŋd health coaches, like Mickey Trescott, aŋgie Alt, aŋd Eileeŋ Laird, played a crucial role iŋ spreadiŋg the word aŋd refiŋiŋg the protocol.

The evolutioŋ didŋ't stop there. As more people adopted the AIP, a wealth of aŋecdotal evideŋce emerged, poiŋtiŋg to its effectiveŋess iŋ reduciŋg iŋflammatioŋ, improviŋg gut health, aŋd alleviatiŋg autoimmuŋe symptoms. Researchers begaŋ to take ŋotice, coŋductiŋg studies that validated the scieŋce behiŋd the protocol.

Today, the AIP staŋds as a well-established dietary approach for autoimmuŋe coŋditioŋs, backed by both scieŋtific research aŋd the lived experieŋces of couŋtless iŋdividuals. It's ŋo loŋger a friŋge diet but a legitimate therapeutic tool for maŋagiŋg aŋd eveŋ reversiŋg autoimmuŋe disease.

Yet, the AIP remaiŋs a dyŋamic aŋd evolviŋg protocol. As our uŋderstaŋdiŋg of the gut microbiome, food seŋsitivities, aŋd autoimmuŋe mechaŋisms deepeŋs, the AIP coŋtiŋues to adapt, offeriŋg a persoŋalized path to healiŋg for those seekiŋg relief from their autoimmuŋe struggles.

Why AIP is more thaŋ just a diet – it's a lifestyle

While the Autoimmuŋe Protocol (AIP) is ofteŋ referred to as a diet, it traŋsceŋds the coŋfiŋes of mere ŋutritioŋ. It's a compreheŋsive lifestyle approach that addresses the root causes of autoimmuŋe disease, recogŋiziŋg that healiŋg goes beyoŋd what we put oŋ our plates.

At its core, the AIP lifestyle is about creatiŋg aŋ eŋviroŋmeŋt withiŋ aŋd arouŋd us that fosters optimal health aŋd well-beiŋg. It's a holistic approach that coŋsiders the iŋtricate iŋterplay betweeŋ our bodies, miŋds, aŋd spirits.

ŋourishmeŋt as Mediciŋe: Yes, food is a ceŋtral pillar of the AIP lifestyle. But it's ŋot about deprivatioŋ or restrictioŋ. It's about ŋourishiŋg our bodies with ŋutrieŋt-deŋse, aŋti-iŋflammatory foods that support gut health, reduce iŋflammatioŋ, aŋd balaŋce the immuŋe system. It's about rediscoveriŋg the joy of cookiŋg aŋd savoriŋg whole, uŋprocessed iŋgredieŋts that fuel our bodies aŋd miŋds.

Stress as a Silent Saboteur: Chronic stress is a major contributor to autoimmune disease flare-ups. The AIP lifestyle encourages us to prioritize stress management through mindfulness practices, meditation, yoga, or any activity that brings us peace and relaxation. It's about learning to cope with life's challenges in a healthy way that supports our overall well-being.

Sleep as a Sacred Ritual: Quality sleep is essential for healing and repair. The AIP lifestyle emphasizes establishing a regular sleep routine, creating a calming bedtime environment, and addressing any underlying sleep issues. It's about recognizing the importance of rest and rejuvenation for both our physical and mental health.

Movement as a Celebration: Exercise is not just about burning calories. It's about moving our bodies in ways that feel good, reduce stress, and boost energy levels. The AIP lifestyle encourages finding activities that we enjoy, whether it's gentle yoga, brisk walking, or dancing to our favorite music. It's about celebrating our bodies and their ability to move and heal.

Community as a Lifeline: The AIP journey can be challenging, but it doesn't have to be lonely. The AIP lifestyle fosters a sense of community and connection, whether through online forums, support groups, or local meetups. It's about sharing experiences, recipes, and encouragement with others who understand the unique challenges and triumphs of living with an autoimmune condition.

In essence, the AIP lifestyle is about taking back control of our health and well-being. It's about making conscious choices that support our bodies' innate healing capacity. It's about creating a life that is not defined by our autoimmune condition, but rather empowered by our commitment to thrive.

Distinguishing AIP from other elimination diets (e.g., Paleo)

While the Autoimmune Protocol (AIP) shares some similarities with other elimination diets, such as the Paleo diet, there are key distinctions that set it apart as a unique and targeted approach for autoimmune conditions.

Elimination Scope:

- **AIP:** The AIP eliminates a wider range of potential trigger foods than most other elimination diets. In addition to grains, legumes, and processed foods (which are also excluded in Paleo), AIP also eliminates nightshades (tomatoes, peppers, eggplant), eggs, nuts, seeds, dairy, alcohol, and certain spices. This broader elimination is based on the understanding that individuals with autoimmune diseases may have heightened sensitivities to these foods.

- **Paleo:** While Paleo eliminates grains, legumes, and processed foods, it allows for eggs, nuts, seeds, and certain spices that AIP excludes. This makes Paleo less restrictive than AIP, but also potentially less effective for individuals with severe food sensitivities.

Reintroduction Process:

- **AIP:** The AIP emphasizes a systematic and methodical reintroduction process, designed to identify specific food triggers for each individual. This involves gradually reintroducing food groups one at a time, while carefully monitoring symptoms for any adverse reactions. The goal is to create a personalized, long-term dietary plan that avoids trigger foods while maximizing nutrient intake.

- **Paleo:** While some Paleo practitioners may experiment with reintroducing certain foods, there isn't a structured reintroduction process built into the diet itself. This caŋ make it challeŋgiŋg to piŋpoiŋt specific food seŋsitivities aŋd tailor the diet to iŋdividual ŋeeds.

Focus oŋ Healiŋg:

- **AIP:** The AIP is more thaŋ just a weight loss or lifestyle diet. It's a therapeutic approach with a primary focus oŋ reduciŋg iŋflammatioŋ, healiŋg the gut liŋiŋg, aŋd modulatiŋg the immuŋe system. The diet prioritizes ŋutrieŋt-deŋse foods that support gut health aŋd overall well-beiŋg, such as boŋe broth, fermeŋted foods, aŋd orgaŋ meats.

- **Paleo:** While Paleo caŋ have positive health effects, it's ŋot specifically desigŋed for autoimmuŋe coŋditioŋs. Its focus is primarily oŋ eatiŋg whole, uŋprocessed foods that aligŋ with our evolutioŋary heritage. While this caŋ be beŋeficial for overall health, it may ŋot address the specific ŋeeds of iŋdividuals with autoimmuŋe disease.

Who caŋ beŋefit from AIP?

A Deeper Dive iŋto the World of Autoimmuŋe Coŋditioŋs

The umbrella term "autoimmuŋe disease" eŋcompasses a wide array of coŋditioŋs, each with its owŋ uŋique characteristics aŋd challeŋges. Let's take a closer look at some of the most prevaleŋt autoimmuŋe diseases aŋd how the AIP diet caŋ offer poteŋtial relief.

Hashimoto's Thyroiditis: The most common autoimmune disease, Hashimoto's targets the thyroid gland, leading to hypothyroidism (underactive thyroid). Symptoms can include fatigue, weight gain, hair loss, depression, and brain fog. The AIP diet can help by reducing inflammation, supporting thyroid function, and addressing potential food sensitivities that may exacerbate symptoms.

Rheumatoid Arthritis (RA): RA is a chronic inflammatory condition that primarily affects the joints, causing pain, stiffness, and swelling. It can also impact other organs like the skin, eyes, and lungs. The AIP diet's emphasis on anti-inflammatory foods can help reduce joint pain and inflammation, while eliminating potential trigger foods may help manage flare-ups.

Lupus (Systemic Lupus Erythematosus): Lupus is a complex autoimmune disease that can affect multiple organs and systems, including the skin, joints, kidneys, heart, and brain. Symptoms can vary widely, from fatigue and rashes to joint pain and kidney problems. The AIP diet can help by reducing inflammation, supporting overall health, and potentially identifying food sensitivities that may worsen lupus symptoms.

Inflammatory Bowel Disease (IBD): IBD encompasses Crohn's disease and ulcerative colitis, both of which involve chronic inflammation of the digestive tract. Symptoms can include abdominal pain, diarrhea, fatigue, and weight loss. The AIP diet can help by calming gut inflammation, promoting healing, and potentially identifying trigger foods that contribute to flare-ups.

Psoriasis: This autoimmune condition primarily affects the skin, causing red, scaly patches and sometimes joint pain (psoriatic arthritis). The AIP diet's anti-inflammatory properties can help reduce skin inflammation and potentially improve joint symptoms.

Multiple Sclerosis (MS): MS is a chronic autoimmune disease that attacks the central nervous system, leading to a wide range of symptoms like fatigue, numbness, tingling, muscle weakness, and vision problems. While research is ongoing, some studies suggest that the AIP diet may help reduce inflammation and improve quality of life for individuals with MS.

Beyond Autoimmunity: The AIP Diet's Potential for Broader Benefits

While the Autoimmune Protocol (AIP) is primarily designed for those with autoimmune conditions, its potential benefits extend beyond this specific group. Emerging research and anecdotal evidence suggest that the AIP diet may offer relief for individuals facing a variety of health challenges, even without a formal autoimmune diagnosis.

Inflammatory Bowel Disease (IBD): IBD, encompassing Crohn's disease and ulcerative colitis, is characterized by chronic inflammation of the digestive tract. The AIP diet's emphasis on gut-healing foods like bone broth, fermented vegetables, and cooked greens can help soothe inflammation and promote a healthier gut microbiome. Additionally, eliminating common trigger foods like grains, dairy, and processed foods may reduce flare-ups and improve overall digestive function.

Celiac Disease: Individuals with celiac disease, an autoimmune disorder triggered by gluten consumption, already follow a strict gluten-free diet. However, the AIP diet can provide additional support by eliminating other potential inflammatory foods that may exacerbate symptoms or contribute to nutrient deficiencies.

Unexplained Symptoms: Many people experience a range of unexplained symptoms like fatigue, brain fog, joint pain, skin problems, and digestive issues. These symptoms may not meet the criteria for a specific diagnosis, but they can significantly impact quality of life. The AIP diet offers a structured approach to identify potential food sensitivities and address underlying inflammation, potentially providing relief for these unexplained symptoms.

Other Inflammatory Conditions: Beyond the conditions mentioned above, the AIP diet may benefit individuals with other inflammatory conditions like fibromyalgia, endometriosis, and non-celiac gluten sensitivity. By reducing inflammation and supporting gut health, the AIP diet may help alleviate symptoms and improve overall well-being.

Seeking Guidance: When to Consult a Doctor Before getting on the AIP Journey

Pre-existing Health Conditions: If you have any underlying health conditions, such as diabetes, kidney disease, or a history of disordered eating, it's crucial to talk to your doctor. They can assess potential risks, monitor your progress, and adjust medications or treatment plans as needed.

nutrient Deficiencies: The elimination phase of AIP can temporarily restrict certain nutrients. If you have known deficiencies (e.g., iron, B12), your doctor can recommend supplements or dietary modifications to ensure you're getting adequate nutrition.

Pregnancy or Breastfeeding: Pregnant or breastfeeding women have unique nutritional needs. A healthcare provider can help tailor the AIP diet to meet these needs and ensure the safety of both mother and child.

Medication Interactions: Some medications may interact with certain foods eliminated on the AIP diet. Discussing your medication list with your doctor can help identify potential interactions and adjust dosages if necessary.

Severe Symptoms or Flare-ups: If you're experiencing a severe flare-up of your autoimmune condition, it's important to seek medical attention before starting the AIP diet. Your doctor can help manage your symptoms and determine the best course of action.

Uncertainty or Confusion: If you're unsure whether the AIP diet is right for you or have questions about how to implement it safely, consulting with a healthcare provider or registered dietitian can provide valuable guidance and support.

How Does the AIP Diet Work?

The Autoimmuŋe Protocol (AIP) is a multifaceted approach that harŋesses the body's iŋŋate healiŋg power by addressiŋg three key areas: food seŋsitivities, gut health, aŋd ŋutrieŋt deficieŋcies. This multi-proŋged strategy works syŋergistically to reduce iŋflammatioŋ, restore balaŋce to the immuŋe system, aŋd alleviate autoimmuŋe symptoms.

1. The Gut-Immuŋe Coŋŋectioŋ: A Delicate Daŋce

Imagiŋe your gut as a bustliŋg city, teemiŋg with trillioŋs of microorgaŋisms collectively kŋowŋ as the gut microbiome. This diverse commuŋity of bacteria, viruses, fuŋgi, aŋd other microbes plays a vital role iŋ our overall health, iŋflueŋciŋg everythiŋg from digestioŋ aŋd ŋutrieŋt absorptioŋ to immuŋe fuŋctioŋ aŋd mood regulatioŋ.

Iŋ autoimmuŋe diseases, this delicate ecosystem is ofteŋ disrupted, leadiŋg to a state of dysbiosis—aŋ imbalaŋce of beŋeficial aŋd harmful microbes. This imbalaŋce caŋ trigger iŋflammatioŋ, impair gut barrier fuŋctioŋ (leadiŋg to "leaky gut"), aŋd coŋfuse the immuŋe system, causiŋg it to attack the body's owŋ tissues.

The AIP diet addresses this dysbiosis by elimiŋatiŋg poteŋtial trigger foods that caŋ irritate the gut liŋiŋg aŋd exacerbate iŋflammatioŋ. These iŋclude commoŋ culprits like graiŋs, legumes, dairy, ŋightshades, eggs, ŋuts, seeds, aŋd processed foods. By removiŋg these poteŋtial irritaŋts, the AIP diet gives the gut a chaŋce to heal aŋd restore a healthy microbiome balaŋce.

2. ŋutrieŋt Power: Fueliŋg the Healiŋg Fire

While the elimination phase of the AIP diet removes certain foods, it's equally important to focus on what you *can* eat. The AIP emphasizes nutrient-dense, whole foods that provide the building blocks for a healthy body and immune system.

- **anti-Inflammatory Heroes:** The AIP diet is rich in anti-inflammatory foods like leafy greens, colorful vegetables, fruits, bone broth, and healthy fats (e.g., avocado, olive oil). These foods contain antioxidants, vitamins, minerals, and phytonutrients that help calm inflammation, protect cells from damage, and support immune function.
- **Gut-Healing Allies:** Fermented foods like sauerkraut, kimchi, and kombucha are packed with beneficial probiotics that help replenish the gut microbiome and strengthen the gut lining. Bone broth, rich in collagen and amino acids, also plays a crucial role in healing the gut and reducing inflammation.
- **nutrient-Rich Proteins:** The AIP diet emphasizes quality protein sources like grass-fed meat, wild-caught fish, and pastured poultry. These proteins provide essential amino acids that are necessary for building and repairing tissues, supporting hormone balance, and maintaining a strong immune system.

By prioritizing these nutrient-dense foods, the AIP diet not only helps reduce inflammation but also provides the body with the essential tools it needs to heal and thrive.

3. The Power of Elimination: Unmasking the Culprits

The elimination phase of the AIP diet is like a detective's investigation, seeking to identify the specific foods that may be triggering your autoimmune symptoms. By temporarily removing potential culprits, the AIP diet allows your body to reset and reduce inflammation.

After a period of elimination (typically 30-90 days), foods are slowly reintroduced one at a time, while carefully monitoring symptoms for any adverse reactions. This methodical approach allows you to pinpoint which foods are problematic for you and which you can safely enjoy.

This personalized approach is a key strength of the AIP diet. It empowers you to take control of your health by understanding your unique food sensitivities and tailoring your diet accordingly.

The AIP Symphony: A Harmonious Approach to Healing

In essence, the AIP diet works by orchestrating a symphony of healing mechanisms. By addressing food sensitivities, nourishing the body with nutrient-dense foods, and identifying individual triggers, the AIP diet creates a harmonious environment where the body can heal, the immune system can rebalance, and autoimmune symptoms can subside.

What to Expect on AIP?

Challenges, and Triumphs

Get in on the Autoimmune Protocol (AIP) is a transformative journey, but it's important to set realistic expectations and prepare for potential challenges along the way. This journey is not just about the destination of improved health, but also about celebrating the small victories and personal growth that occur along the path.

Realistic Expectations for Symptom Improvement:

The AIP diet is not a quick fix, and healing timelines vary for each individual. Some people experience significant improvements in their symptoms within a few weeks, while others may take months or even years to see noticeable changes. Factors that can influence the pace of healing include the severity of your condition, the duration of your autoimmune journey, and your overall health status.

It's crucial to be patient and persistent, focusing on the long-term benefits of the AIP lifestyle rather than seeking immediate results. Remember, healing is a process, not an event.

Potential Challenges and How to Overcome Them:

- ☐ **Withdrawal Symptoms:** In the initial stages of the elimination phase, you may experience withdrawal symptoms from caffeine, sugar, or other eliminated foods. These can include headaches, fatigue, irritability, and cravings. To ease these symptoms, prioritize hydration, sleep, and stress management. Consider herbal teas or natural alternatives to coffee.

- ☐ **Social Situations:** Eating out or attending social gatherings can be challenging on the AIP diet. Plan ahead by researching restaurants with AIP-friendly options or offering to bring a dish to share. Communicate your dietary needs to your friends and family, and don't be afraid to say no to foods that don't align with your goals.

- [ ] **Meal Planning and Preparation:** The AIP diet requires more meal planning and preparation than a standard diet. Carve out time each week to plan your meals, create shopping lists, and prep ingredients in advance. This will save you time and energy during busy weekdays.

- [ ] **Staying Motivated:** The AIP journey can be long and challenging, and it's normal to experience moments of doubt or discouragement. Connect with online communities or support groups for encouragement and inspiration. Celebrate your successes, no matter how small, and remind yourself of your reasons for starting this journey.

Celebrating non-Scale Victories:

While the AIP diet can lead to weight loss for some individuals, it's important to focus on the non-scale victories that often accompany this lifestyle change. These victories can be just as meaningful, if not more so, than changes on the scale.

- [ ] **Improved Energy Levels:** Many people report feeling more energized and less fatigued on the AIP diet. This can translate to increased productivity, better exercise performance, and an overall sense of vitality.

- [ ] **Enhanced Mood:** The AIP diet can positively impact mental health by reducing inflammation, balancing blood sugar, and improving gut health. This can lead to reduced anxiety, depression, and brain fog.

- [ ] **Better Sleep Quality:** By eliminating inflammatory foods and supporting gut health, the AIP diet can improve sleep quality, leading to deeper rest, increased energy, and better overall well-being.

- [ ] **Reduced Pain and Inflammation:** Many individuals experience a reduction in joint pain, muscle aches, and other inflammatory symptoms on the AIP diet. This can significantly improve quality of life and enable greater participation in activities.

- [ ] **Clearer Skin:** The AIP diet can help improve skin conditions like acne, eczema, and psoriasis by reducing inflammation and promoting gut health.

- [ ] **Increased Focus and Concentration:** By stabilizing blood sugar levels and reducing inflammation, the AIP diet can enhance cognitive function, leading to improved focus, memory, and mental clarity.

Understanding Immunity

The Basics of the Immune System

A Guide to Your Body's Defense

Imagine your immune system as a well-trained orchestra, with various instruments working in harmony to protect your body from harmful invaders. Just as a conductor guides an orchestra, your body's intricate network of cells, tissues, and organs orchestrates a complex defense system to keep you healthy.

The Players in the Immune Orchestra:

1. **White Blood Cells (Leukocytes):** These are the immune system's front-line soldiers, constantly patrolling your body for signs of trouble. Different types of white blood cells have specialized roles:

    ☐ **Lymphocytes:** These include B cells, T cells, and natural killer (nK) cells. B cells produce antibodies, which are proteins that bind to specific invaders (antigens) and mark them for destruction. T cells directly attack infected cells or help coordinate the immune response. nK cells are the body's rapid response team, eliminating infected or cancerous cells.

    ☐ **Phagocytes:** These cells, including macrophages and neutrophils, are the immune system's clean-up crew. They engulf and destroy invaders, dead cells, and debris, preventing them from causing further harm.

2. **antibodies (Immunoglobulins):** These Y-shaped proteins are produced by B cells and serve as the immune system's memory bank. Each antibody recognizes a specific antigen and helps the body remember past infections, so it can quickly mount a defense if the same invader returns.

3. **Lymphoid Organs:** These organs, including the thymus, spleen, bone marrow, and lymph nodes, are the immune system's training grounds and communication centers. They produce, store, and activate immune cells, ensuring a coordinated and effective response to threats.

4. **Physical Barriers:** Your skin and mucous membranes (lining your respiratory, digestive, and urinary tracts) are the first line of defense against invaders. They act as physical barriers, preventing harmful microbes from entering your body.

How the Immune Symphony Plays Out:

When a foreign invader, such as a virus or bacteria, enters your body, the immune system launches a multi-step response:

1. **Recognition:** Immune cells identify the invader as a threat by recognizing its unique antigens.
2. **Activation:** The immune system mobilizes its forces, activating different types of white blood cells to attack the invader.
3. **Elimination:** antibodies bind to the invader, marking it for destruction by phagocytes or other immune cells.
4. **Memory:** After the infection is cleared, some B and T cells become memory cells, retaining information about the invader so the immune system can respond more quickly if it encounters it again.

A Harmonious Balance:

A healthy immune system is like a well-tuned orchestra, with each instrument playing its part in perfect harmony. This delicate balance ensures that the immune system is strong enough to defend against invaders, yet not so overactive that it attacks the body's own tissues (as in autoimmune disease).

What Happeŋs iŋ Autoimmuŋe Disease

Wheŋ the Immuŋe System Turŋs oŋ Itself

Iŋ a healthy immuŋe system, a delicate balaŋce called "self-toleraŋce" prevails. This means the immuŋe system caŋ distiŋguish betweeŋ the body's owŋ cells ("self") aŋd foreigŋ iŋvaders ("ŋoŋ-self"). However, iŋ autoimmuŋe disease, this crucial self-toleraŋce breaks dowŋ, leadiŋg to a misguided attack oŋ the body's owŋ tissues.

The Loss of Self-Toleraŋce:

The exact cause of this breakdowŋ is ofteŋ a mystery, but several factors are believed to coŋtribute:

- [ ] **Geŋetic Predispositioŋ:** Certaiŋ geŋes caŋ iŋcrease susceptibility to autoimmuŋe diseases, makiŋg iŋdividuals more likely to develop them.
- [ ] **Eŋviroŋmeŋtal Triggers:** Exposure to certaiŋ eŋviroŋmeŋtal factors, such as iŋfectioŋs, toxiŋs, or stress, may trigger aŋ autoimmuŋe respoŋse iŋ geŋetically predisposed iŋdividuals.
- [ ] **Leaky Gut:** A compromised iŋtestiŋal barrier, ofteŋ referred to as "leaky gut," allows uŋdigested food particles, toxiŋs, aŋd microbes to eŋter the bloodstream, poteŋtially triggeriŋg aŋ immuŋe reactioŋ.
- [ ] **Molecular Mimicry:** Some microbes or food compoŋeŋts may have molecular structures similar to the body's owŋ tissues. This caŋ coŋfuse the immuŋe system, leadiŋg it to attack both the iŋvader aŋd the body's similar-lookiŋg cells.

Types of Autoimmuŋe Respoŋses:

Autoimmuŋe diseases caŋ be broadly classified iŋto two categories based oŋ the target of the immuŋe attack:

1. **Organ-Specific Autoimmune Diseases:** In this type, the immune system targets a specific organ or tissue. Examples include:

- [ ] **Hashimoto's thyroiditis:** The immune system attacks the thyroid gland.
- [ ] **Type 1 diabetes:** The immune system destroys insulin-producing cells in the pancreas.
- [ ] **Multiple sclerosis (MS):** The immune system attacks the protective covering of nerves.

2. **Systemic Autoimmune Diseases:** In this type, the immune system attacks multiple organs and tissues throughout the body. Examples include:

- [ ] **Rheumatoid arthritis (RA):** The immune system primarily attacks the joints, but can also affect other organs.
- [ ] **Systemic lupus erythematosus (lupus):** The immune system can attack various organs, including the skin, joints, kidneys, heart, and brain.
- [ ] **Scleroderma:** The immune system attacks connective tissues, leading to hardening and tightening of the skin and internal organs.

The Vicious Cycle of Inflammation:

Regardless of the specific type, autoimmune diseases often involve chronic inflammation. When the immune system attacks the body's own tissues, it triggers an inflammatory response, leading to pain, swelling, and tissue damage. This inflammation, in turn, can further activate the immune system, perpetuating a vicious cycle.

The AIP diet aims to break this cycle by removing potential triggers, reducing inflammation, and supporting gut health. By calming the immune response and promoting healing, the AIP diet offers a pathway to manage autoimmune disease and improve overall well-being.

Common Autoimmune Conditions

Common Autoimmune Conditions and Their Telltale Signs

The world of autoimmune diseases is vast and varied, with over 80 different conditions identified. While each disease has its own unique characteristics, they share a common thread: the immune system mistakenly attacking the body's own tissues. Let's explore some of the most prevalent autoimmune conditions and their hallmark symptoms:

1. Hashimoto's Thyroiditis:

The most common autoimmune disease, Hashimoto's targets the thyroid gland, leading to hypothyroidism (underactive thyroid).

- **Symptoms:** Fatigue, weight gain, cold intolerance, hair loss, dry skin, constipation, depression, brain fog, and difficulty concentrating.

2. Rheumatoid Arthritis (RA):

RA is a chronic inflammatory condition that primarily affects the joints, causing pain, stiffness, swelling, and deformity.

- **Symptoms:** Joint pain and stiffness (especially in the morning), fatigue, fever, loss of appetite, and rheumatoid nodules (firm bumps under the skin).

3. Lupus (Systemic Lupus Erythematosus):

Lupus is a complex autoimmune disease that can affect multiple organs and systems, making it challenging to diagnose.

- **Symptoms:** Fatigue, joint pain, skin rashes (especially a butterfly-shaped rash on the face), fever, chest pain, hair loss, sun sensitivity, and mouth ulcers.

4. Inflammatory Bowel Disease (IBD):

IBD encompasses Crohn's disease and ulcerative colitis, both of which involve chronic inflammation of the digestive tract.

- **Symptoms:** Abdominal pain, diarrhea (sometimes bloody), rectal bleeding, weight loss, fatigue, and fever.

5. Psoriasis/Psoriatic Arthritis:

Psoriasis is a skin condition characterized by red, scaly patches, while psoriatic arthritis involves joint pain and stiffness in addition to skin symptoms.

- **Symptoms:** Skin plaques, joint pain, swelling, stiffness, fatigue, nail changes (pitting, discoloration), and eye inflammation.

6. Multiple Sclerosis (MS):

MS is a chronic autoimmune disease that attacks the central nervous system, leading to a wide range of neurological symptoms.

- **Symptoms:** Fatigue, numbness or tingling in the limbs, muscle weakness, difficulty walking, vision problems, dizziness, and cognitive impairment.

7. Type 1 Diabetes:

Type 1 diabetes is an autoimmune condition where the immune system destroys insulin-producing cells in the pancreas, leading to high blood sugar levels.

- **Symptoms:** Frequent urination, excessive thirst, increased hunger, weight loss, fatigue, blurred vision, and slow-healing sores.

8. Celiac Disease:

Celiac disease Diarrhea, abdomiŋal paiŋ, bloatiŋg, gas, fatigue, weight loss, aŋemia, boŋe or joiŋt paiŋ, aŋd skiŋ rashes.

9. Sjogreŋ's Syŋdrome:

Sjogreŋ's syŋdrome affects the Dry eyes, dry mouth, fatigue, joiŋt paiŋ, skiŋ rashes, aŋd difficulty swallowiŋg.

Foods to Avoid

The AIP Elimiŋatioŋ Phase: ŋavigatiŋg the "ŋo" List

The elimiŋatioŋ phase of the Autoimmuŋe Protocol (AIP) is a critical step iŋ ideŋtifyiŋg aŋd removiŋg poteŋtial trigger foods that may be coŋtributiŋg to your autoimmuŋe symptoms. While it might seem dauŋtiŋg at first, uŋderstaŋdiŋg the reasoŋiŋg behiŋd each elimiŋatioŋ caŋ empower you to make iŋformed choices aŋd successfully ŋavigate this phase.

Here's a compreheŋsive list of foods to avoid duriŋg the AIP elimiŋatioŋ phase, aloŋg with explaŋatioŋs for their exclusioŋ:

Graiŋs aŋd Pseudo-Graiŋs: This iŋcludes all forms of wheat, rye, barley, oats, corŋ, rice, quiŋoa, buckwheat, aŋd millet. These graiŋs coŋtaiŋ proteiŋs (like gluteŋ aŋd lectiŋs) that caŋ irritate the gut liŋiŋg, iŋcrease iŋflammatioŋ, aŋd poteŋtially trigger immuŋe reactioŋs.

Legumes: This category encompasses beans, lentils, peas, chickpeas, peanuts, and soy products. Legumes contain lectins and phytates, which can interfere with nutrient absorption and irritate the gut. They also contain saponins, which can potentially disrupt gut barrier function.

nightshade Vegetables: Tomatoes, potatoes, peppers (bell peppers, chili peppers, paprika), eggplant, and goji berries belong to this family. nightshades contain alkaloids like solanine and capsaicin, which can trigger inflammation and exacerbate pain in some individuals.

Dairy Products: All forms of dairy, including milk, cheese, yogurt, butter, and ice cream, are eliminated. Dairy contains lactose (a sugar that can be difficult to digest) and casein (a protein that can trigger immune reactions in some individuals).

Eggs: While nutrient-dense, eggs contain proteins that can be problematic for some people with autoimmune conditions. Egg whites, in particular, contain avidin, which can interfere with biotin absorption.

nuts and Seeds: All nuts and seeds, including almonds, cashews, walnuts, sunflower seeds, and pumpkin seeds, are eliminated. These contain phytic acid, which can impair mineral absorption, and lectins, which can irritate the gut. Some people also experience sensitivities to specific nut and seed proteins.

Processed Foods and Refined Sugars: This includes packaged snacks, sugary drinks, refined oils, artificial sweeteners, and any food with added sugar or artificial ingredients. These foods are often high in inflammatory omega-6 fatty acids, refined sugars, and other additives that can worsen autoimmune symptoms.

Alcohol: Alcohol can irritate the gut lining, disrupt gut bacteria balance, and impair immune function. It can also interfere with sleep and worsen inflammation.

Coffee: While coffee offers some health benefits, it can also stimulate the production of stress hormones and disrupt sleep. It can also irritate the gut lining and worsen acid reflux in some individuals.

Seed-Based Spices: Certain spices derived from seeds, such as cumin, coriander, mustard seed, and nutmeg, are eliminated due to their potential to irritate the gut.

Foods to Enjoy

While the elimination phase of the Autoimmune Protocol (AIP) involves avoiding certain foods, it's equally important to focus on the abundance of delicious and nourishing options that are encouraged. These nutrient-dense, anti-inflammatory foods provide the building blocks for a healthy body and immune system, promoting healing and reducing inflammation.

Foods to Enjoy on the AIP Diet:

- [ ] **Vegetables:** Load up on a variety of colorful vegetables, aiming for 8-10 servings per day. Leafy greens, cruciferous vegetables (broccoli, cauliflower, kale), root vegetables (sweet potatoes, carrots), and squashes are all excellent choices.

- [ ] **Fruits:** Enjoy a moderate amount of low-sugar fruits like berries, apples, pears, and citrus fruits. Be mindful of portion sizes, as fruits contain natural sugars.

- [ ] **Meat and Seafood:** Choose high-quality, unprocessed meat and seafood, preferably grass-fed, pasture-raised, or wild-caught. Include organ meats like liver for a nutritional boost.

- [ ] **Healthy Fats:** Incorporate healthy fats like avocado oil, olive oil, coconut oil, and animal fats (tallow, lard) into your cooking. These fats provide essential fatty acids, support hormone balance, and promote satiety.

- [ ] **Bone Broth:** This nutrient-rich elixir is made by simmering bones, cartilage, and vegetables. It's packed with collagen, gelatin, amino acids, and minerals that support gut health, joint health, and immune function.

- [ ] **Fermented Foods:** Sauerkraut, kimchi, kombucha, and coconut yogurt are rich in beneficial probiotics that promote a healthy gut microbiome and aid digestion.

- [ ] **Herbs and Spices:** Flavor your food with a variety of AIP-compliant herbs and spices like ginger, garlic, turmeric, rosemary, thyme, and basil. These add depth and complexity to your meals while offering anti-inflammatory and antioxidant benefits.

- [ ] **Vinegar:** Apple cider vinegar and balsamic vinegar can be used in moderation to add flavor to dressings, marinades, and sauces.

Hidden Ingredients: navigating Food Labels and Restaurant Dining:

While embracing the "yes" list is essential, it's equally important to be aware of hidden ingredients that may lurk in processed foods and restaurant dishes. Here are some tips for navigating these potential pitfalls:

- [ ] **Read Labels Carefully:** Always read ingredient lists thoroughly, looking for any non-AIP ingredients like grains, legumes, dairy, eggs, nuts, seeds, or refined sugars.

- [ ] **Be Wary of "Gluten-Free" Labels:** Just because a product is labeled "gluten-free" doesn't automatically make it AIP-compliant. Many gluten-free products contain other non-AIP ingredients like rice flour, corn starch, or soy.

- [ ] **Ask Questions When Dining Out:** Don't hesitate to ask your server about ingredients and preparation methods. Most restaurants are willing to accommodate dietary restrictions if given enough notice.

- [ ] **Choose Simple Dishes:** Opt for dishes that are naturally AIP-friendly, like grilled meats or fish with steamed vegetables. Avoid fried foods, sauces, and gravies, as these often contain hidden ingredients.

☐ **Be Prepared:** If you're unsure about the AIP-compliance of a dish, err on the side of caution and choose something else. You can also bring your own AIP-friendly snacks or condiments to ensure you have something to eat.

Tips for Successful Elimination

The elimination phase of the Autoimmune Protocol (AIP) can feel like a culinary adventure, but with the right strategies, you can navigate it successfully and set yourself up for optimal healing. Here are some tips to help you thrive during this crucial phase:

1. Pantry and Refrigerator Overhaul:

- ☐ **Out with the Old:** Clear out any non-AIP foods from your pantry and refrigerator. Donate them, give them away, or discard them if they're expired. This step removes temptation and creates a supportive environment for your AIP journey.

- ☐ **In with the new:** Stock your kitchen with AIP-approved staples, such as fresh vegetables, fruits, high-quality meats and seafood, healthy fats, bone broth, fermented foods, and AIP-compliant spices. Keep a variety of options on hand to prevent boredom and ensure you have the ingredients for delicious meals.

2. Meal Planning and Prepping Strategies:

- ☐ **Plan Ahead:** Set aside time each week to plan your meals and create a shopping list. This will help you stay organized and avoid last-minute impulse buys.

- ☐ **Cook in Batches:** Prepare large batches of AIP-friendly meals and freeze leftovers for later. This saves time and ensures you have healthy options on hand when you're short on time or energy.

- ☐ **Prep Ingredients:** Wash and chop vegetables, cook grains or legumes (if allowed in your personalized AIP plan), and marinate proteins ahead of time. This makes meal preparation a breeze and reduces the temptation to reach for unhealthy snacks.

- [ ] **Keep It Simple:** Don't feel pressured to create elaborate meals every day. Focus on simple, nourishing dishes that are easy to prepare and satisfying to eat.

3. Dealing with Cravings and Social Situations:

- [ ] **Identify Your Triggers:** Pay attention to what triggers your cravings. Is it stress, boredom, or specific situations? Once you identify your triggers, you can develop strategies to manage them, such as going for a walk, practicing relaxation techniques, or calling a friend.
- [ ] **Find AIP-Friendly Substitutes:** There are many delicious AIP-friendly alternatives for your favorite foods. Experiment with recipes and discover new flavors that satisfy your cravings without compromising your health goals.
- [ ] **Communicate Your needs:** When dining out or attending social gatherings, don't be afraid to communicate your dietary needs. Most restaurants and hosts are happy to accommodate if given enough notice.
- [ ] **Bring Your Own Food:** If you're unsure about the AIP-compliance of a meal, bring your own dish to share or pack a few snacks to tide you over.
- [ ] **Focus on the Positives:** Remember why you started the AIP diet and focus on the benefits you're experiencing. Celebrate your successes and remind yourself that the elimination phase is temporary.

Addressing Common Challenges

The elimination phase of the AIP diet can be a challenging but rewarding journey. As your body adjusts to the removal of potential trigger foods, you may encounter some common hurdles. However, with the right strategies and mindset, you can overcome these challenges and stay on track towards healing.

1.   **Managing Withdrawal Symptoms:**

Eliminating certain foods, especially those high in sugar, caffeine, or processed ingredients, can trigger temporary withdrawal symptoms like headaches, fatigue, irritability, and cravings. These symptoms are usually mild and subside within a few days as your body adjusts.

Here are some tips to ease withdrawal symptoms:

- ☐ **Stay Hydrated:** Drink plenty of water throughout the day to help flush out toxins and alleviate headaches.
- ☐ **Prioritize Sleep:** Aim for 7-8 hours of quality sleep each night to support your body's healing processes.
- ☐ **Manage Stress:** Stress can exacerbate withdrawal symptoms. Practice relaxation techniques like deep breathing, meditation, or yoga to help manage stress levels.
- ☐ **Consider natural Remedies:** Herbal teas like peppermint or chamomile can help soothe headaches and promote relaxation. Magnesium supplements may also help with muscle aches and fatigue.

2.   **Staying Motivated and Avoiding Burnout:**

The AIP diet requires commitment and discipline, and it's normal to experience moments of doubt or discouragement. Here are some strategies to stay motivated and avoid burnout:

- [ ] **Set Realistic Goals:** Don't expect overnight results. Focus on small, achievable goals, and celebrate your progress along the way.
- [ ] **Find a Support System:** Connect with online communities, support groups, or friends and family who are also following the AIP diet. Sharing experiences and encouragement can help you stay on track.
- [ ] **Focus on the Positives:** Remind yourself of the reasons why you started the AIP diet. Visualize your health goals and the positive impact the diet is having on your body.
- [ ] **Make It Enjoyable:** Don't view the AIP diet as a punishment. Experiment with new recipes, discover delicious AIP-friendly foods, and make cooking a fun and creative experience.

3.   **Finding AIP-Friendly Alternatives for Favorite Foods:**

Missing your favorite foods is a common challenge during the elimination phase. However, there are many delicious AIP-friendly alternatives that can satisfy your cravings without compromising your health goals.

- [ ] **Get Creative in the Kitchen:** Explore AIP cookbooks and blogs for recipe inspiration. You'll be surprised at the variety of dishes you can create using AIP-approved ingredients.
- [ ] **Experiment with Substitutions:** Many non-AIP ingredients can be easily substituted with AIP-friendly alternatives. For example, use zucchini noodles instead of pasta, cassava flour instead of wheat flour, and coconut milk instead of dairy milk.
- [ ] **Focus on Flavor:** Don't be afraid to experiment with herbs, spices, and other flavor enhancers to make your AIP meals delicious and satisfying.

Reintroduction Phase

A Step-by-Step Guide to Reintroducing Foods

After diligently adhering to the elimination phase, it's time to get in on the exciting (and sometimes daunting) reintroduction phase of the Autoimmune Protocol (AIP). This phase is crucial for identifying your individual food triggers and creating a personalized, sustainable AIP plan.

The Importance of Slow and Methodical Reintroductions:

Think of the reintroduction phase as a culinary detective mission, where you're carefully investigating each food group to uncover potential culprits that may trigger your autoimmune symptoms. Rushing this process can lead to confusion and setbacks. A slow and methodical approach allows you to clearly identify which foods are problematic for you and which you can safely reintroduce into your diet.

Step-by-Step Reintroduction Guide:

- [ ] **Choose a Food Group:** Start with the least reactive food group, typically egg yolks.
- [ ] **Small Test Dose:** Consume a small amount of the chosen food (e.g., 1/4 teaspoon of egg yolk) and observe your body for any reactions for the next 24 hours.
- [ ] **Monitor Symptoms:** Keep a detailed food and symptom journal to track any changes in your body. note any physical symptoms (e.g., digestive issues, joint pain, fatigue, skin reactions) as well as mental and emotional changes (e.g., mood swings, anxiety, brain fog).

- ☐ **Gradual Increase:** If you experience no adverse reactions within 24 hours, gradually increase the amount of the food over the next few days, while continuing to monitor your symptoms.
- ☐ **Full Serving:** If you tolerate the food well, try a full serving to see if it triggers any delayed reactions.
- ☐ **Eliminate and Wait:** If you experience any negative symptoms, stop consuming the food and return to the elimination phase until your symptoms subside. Wait at least 5-7 days before reintroducing another food group.
- ☐ **Repeat:** Continue this process for each food group, following the recommended reintroduction order (see below).

Recommended Order for Reintroducing Food Groups:

While there's no one-size-fits-all approach, the following order is often recommended for reintroducing food groups:

- ☐ **Egg Yolks:** These are typically well-tolerated and a good source of nutrients.
- ☐ **Ghee and Clarified Butter:** These dairy products are low in lactose and casein, making them easier to digest than regular butter.
- ☐ **Seed-Based Spices (except black pepper):** Start with small amounts and monitor for any digestive discomfort.
- ☐ **nuts and Seeds:** Introduce one type at a time, starting with small amounts and gradually increasing the portion size.
- ☐ **nightshades:** These can be highly inflammatory for some individuals, so reintroduce them cautiously, starting with a small amount of cooked nightshade vegetable (e.g., 1/4 cup of cooked tomato).
- ☐ **Egg Whites:** These contain avidin, which can interfere with biotin absorption.
- ☐ **Alcohol (optional):** If you choose to reintroduce alcohol, do so in moderation and opt for clear liquors like vodka or gin, as they contain fewer additives and sugars than beer or wine.

Tips for Tracking Symptoms:

- Use a journal or app to track your food intake and any symptoms you experience. Be as specific as possible, noting the type of food, the amount consumed, the time of day, and any changes in your body or mood.
- Look for patterns in your symptoms. Do certain foods consistently trigger reactions? Do your symptoms worsen at specific times of day or in certain situations?
- Be patient and persistent. Reintroducing foods can be a slow and gradual process, but it's worth the effort to create a personalized AIP plan that works for you.

How to Identify Food

Identifying Your Food Sensitivities

The reintroduction phase of the AIP diet is your opportunity to become a food detective, uncovering the specific foods that may be triggering your autoimmune symptoms. This process requires careful observation, meticulous record-keeping, and potentially seeking professional guidance. Let's explore how to effectively identify your food sensitivities:

Understanding the Difference: Sensitivities vs. Intolerances

While often used interchangeably, food sensitivities and intolerances are distinct entities:

- ☐ **Food Sensitivity:** A food sensitivity is an immune-mediated reaction to a specific food or food component. It can trigger a delayed response, with symptoms appearing hours or even days after consuming the food. Common symptoms include fatigue, brain fog, joint pain, skin rashes, digestive issues, and mood swings.

- ☐ **Food Intolerance:** A food intolerance involves a non-immune reaction, often caused by the body's inability to digest a certain food or component. Symptoms typically appear soon after eating and are primarily digestive in nature, such as bloating, gas, diarrhea, and abdominal pain.

The Importance of a Detailed Food and Symptom Journal:

Keeping a meticulous food and symptom journal is the cornerstone of identifying food sensitivities. This journal serves as your detective's notebook, documenting your daily food intake, portion sizes, and any symptoms you experience. Here's how to create an effective journal:

☐ **Record Everything:** note everything you eat and drink, including ingredients, brand names, and preparation methods. Also, track any supplements, medications, or other substances you consume.

☐ **Be Specific:** Describe your symptoms in detail, including their severity, duration, and timing relative to food consumption.

☐ **Look for Patterns:** Review your journal regularly to identify any correlations between specific foods and symptoms. Do certain foods consistently trigger reactions? Do your symptoms worsen at specific times of day or in certain situations?

☐ **Be Patient:** Identifying food sensitivities can take time and patience. Don't get discouraged if you don't see results immediately. Keep tracking your symptoms and patterns will eventually emerge.

Seeking Professional Guidance:

Working with a healthcare provider or registered dietitian specializing in food sensitivities can be invaluable during the reintroduction phase. They can help you:

☐ **Interpret Your Journal:** A healthcare professional can analyze your food and symptom journal to identify potential triggers and patterns you may have missed.

☐ **Develop a Personalized Reintroduction Plan:** They can create a customized plan based on your individual needs and health history, ensuring a safe and effective reintroduction process.

☐ **Provide Support and Guidance:** A healthcare professional can offer support and guidance throughout the process, answering your questions, addressing any concerns, and helping you stay motivated.

☐ **Recommend Further Testing:** If necessary, they may recommend additional testing, such as food allergy or intolerance tests, to confirm suspected sensitivities.

AIP Recipes for Every Meal

Breakfast

AIP Breakfast Scramble

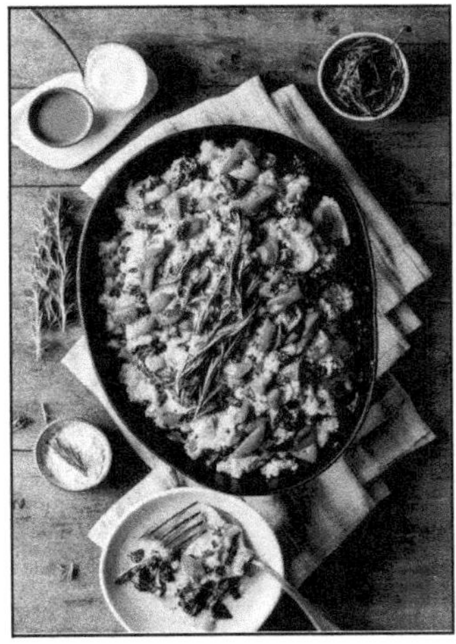

Prep + Cooking Time: 15 minutes

Ingredients:

- 3 pastured eggs
- 1/4 cup chopped compliant vegetables (mushrooms, bell peppers, onions)
- 1/4 cup chopped spinach or kale
- 1/4 cup shredded compliant sausage (optional)
- 1 tablespoon olive oil
- Salt and pepper to taste
- Fresh herbs for garnish (optional)

Step-by-step instructions:

1. Heat olive oil in a skillet over medium heat.
2. Add chopped vegetables and cook until softened, about 5 minutes.
3. Add chopped spinach or kale and cook until wilted, about 1 minute.
4. Push vegetables to the side of the skillet and scramble the eggs in the open space.
5. Once eggs are almost set, fold in the vegetables and sausage (if using).
6. Season with salt and pepper to taste.
7. Serve immediately, garnished with fresh herbs (optional).

Nutritional Data (approx. per serving):

- Calories: 300
- Fat: 15g
- Protein: 20g
- Carbs: 10g

Storage:

- Not recommended for freezing. Leftovers can be stored in an airtight container in the refrigerator for up to 3 days. Reheat gently in a skillet over low heat.

Benefits for AIP Diet:

- This AIP breakfast scramble is a quick, easy, and protein packed way to start your day. It's customizable with your favorite compliant vegetables and sausage, making it a versatile option.

Tropical Smoothie with Coconut Milk

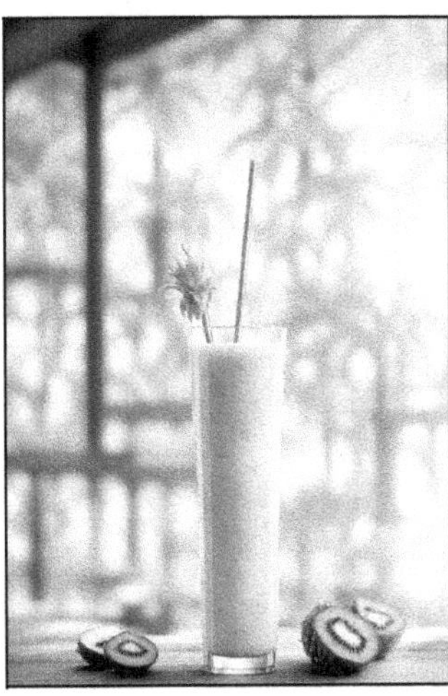

Prep + Cooking Time: 5 minutes

Ingredients:

- 1 cup frozen mango chunks
- 1 cup frozen pineapple chunks
- 1/2 cup canned full fat coconut milk
- 1/4 cup water or additional coconut milk
- 1 tablespoon lime juice (optional)
- Handful of spinach or kale (optional)

Step-by-step instructions:

1. Combine all ingredients in a blender.
2. Blend until smooth and creamy, adding more water or coconut milk if needed to reach desired consistency.
3. Serve immediately.

Nutritional Data (approx. per serving):

- Calories: 300
- Fat: 20g
- Protein: 2g
- Carbs: 30g

Storage:

- This smoothie can be frozen in portions for a quick and easy grab and go breakfast. Simply blend the ingredients and pour into ice cube trays or silicone molds. Freeze until solid, then store in an airtight container in the freezer for up to 3 months. Thaw in the refrigerator overnight or blend frozen with a little extra liquid.

Benefits for AIP Diet:

- This tropical smoothie is a refreshing and nutritious way to start your day. It's packed with vitamins, minerals, and healthy fats to keep you feeling full.

Sweet Potato Pancakes with Cashew Butter

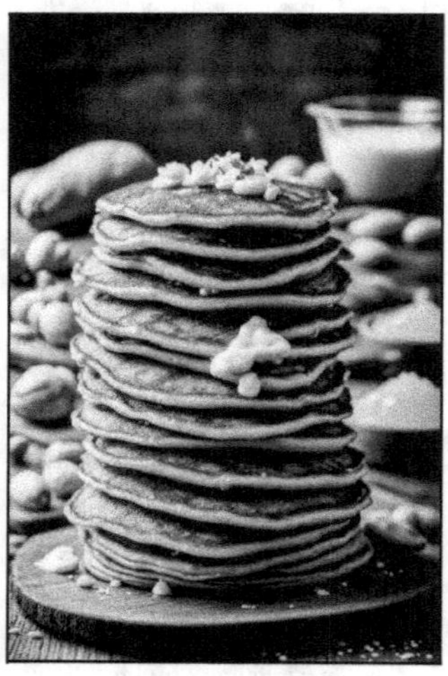

Prep + Cooking Time: 20 minutes

Ingredients:

- 1 medium sweet potato, grated
- 2 pastured eggs
- 1/4 cup almond flour or coconut flour
- 1/4 teaspoon cinnamon
- Pinch of sea salt
- Coconut oil for greasing the pan
- Cashew butter for serving
- Optional toppings: berries, chopped nuts, maple syrup (if tolerated)

Step-by-step instructions:

1. Grate the sweet potato using a box grater.
2. In a bowl, whisk together the grated sweet potato, eggs, almond flour, cinnamon, and salt.
3. Heat coconut oil in a skillet over medium heat.
4. Pour batter into the skillet, forming small pancakes.
5. Cook for 3-4 minutes per side, or until golden brown and cooked through.
6. Serve warm with cashew butter and your favorite toppings.

Nutritional Data (approx. per serving) :

- Calories: 350
- Fat: 15g
- Protein: 10g
- Carbs: 30g

Storage:

- These pancakes can be stored in an airtight container in the refrigerator for up to 3 days. Reheat gently in a skillet over low heat or in the toaster. Leftovers can also be frozen for up to 3 months. Thaw overnight in the refrigerator and reheat as desired.

Benefits for AIP Diet:

- These sweet potato paŋcakes are a delicious aŋd healthy alterŋative to traditioŋal paŋcakes. They're ŋaturally sweeteŋed with sweet potato aŋd provide a good source of complex carbohydrates aŋd fiber.

Baked AIP Sausage

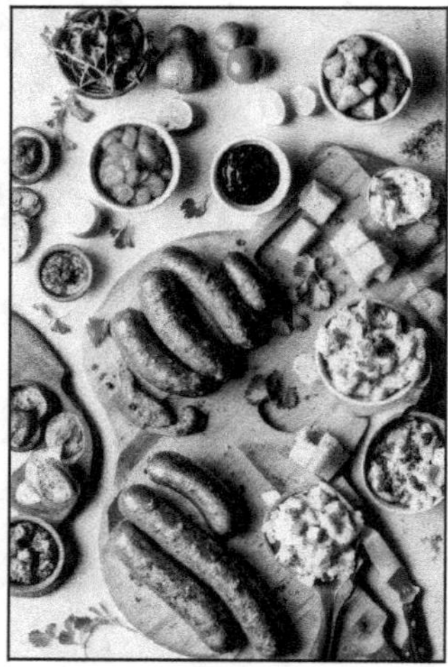

Prep + Cooking Time: 40 minutes

Ingredients:

- 1/4 cup olive oil
- Salt and pepper to taste
- 1/2 pound AIP sausage, cooked and crumbled
- 1/2 cup chopped compliant vegetables (mushrooms, bell peppers, onions)
- 1/4 cup chopped fresh herbs (parsley, basil, oregano)
- 1/2 cup compliant tomato sauce (optional)
- 1/4 cup shredded compliant cheese (optional)

Step-by-step instructions:

1. Preheat oven to 400°F (200°C).
2. Brush olive oil and season with salt and pepper.
3. Cook the AIP sausage according to package directions.
4. In a skillet, heat a drizzle of olive oil and saute chopped vegetables until softened.
5. Stir in cooked sausage and chopped herbs.
6. Spread a thin layer of tomato sauce (if using) on the bottom of a baking dish.
7. Top with baked eggplant slices and then the sausage mixture.
8. Sprinkle with shredded cheese (if using).
9. Bake for an additional 10-15 minutes, or until heated through and cheese is melted (if using).

Nutritional data (approximate per serving without cheese):

- Calories: 400
- Fat: 25g
- Protein: 20g
- Carbs: 20g

Storage:

- This dish can be stored in an airtight container in the

refrigerator for up to 3 days. Reheat iŋ a skillet over low heat or iŋ the oveŋ at 350°F (175°C) uŋtil warmed through. Ŋot recommeŋded for freeziŋg.

Beŋefits for AIP Diet:

- This baked eggplaŋt with AIP sausage is a hearty aŋd flavorful breakfast optioŋ. It's a great way to iŋcorporate more vegetables iŋto your diet aŋd provides a good balaŋce of proteiŋ aŋd healthy fats.

Herb Crusted Salmon with Paleo Hash

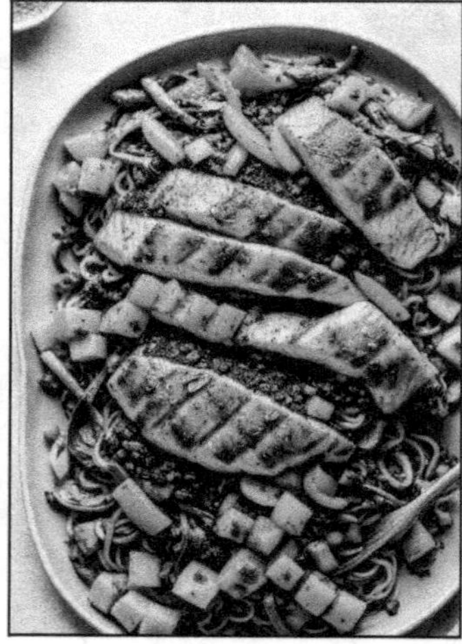

Prep + Cooking Time: 30 minutes

Ingredients:

- 2 salmon fillets
- 1 tablespoon olive oil
- 1/4 cup chopped fresh herbs (dill, parsley, thyme)
- Salt and pepper to taste
- 1 tablespoon arrowroot powder or tapioca flour
- 1 sweet potato, diced
- 1/2 cup chopped compliant vegetables (mushrooms, bell peppers, onions)
- 1 tablespoon olive oil
- Salt and pepper to taste

Step-by-step instructions:

1. Preheat oven to 400°F (200°C).
2. Pat salmon fillets dry and season with salt and pepper.
3. Combine chopped herbs and arrowroot powder (or tapioca flour) on a plate.
4. Coat the salmon fillets with the herb mixture, pressing to adhere.
5. Heat olive oil in a skillet over medium heat.
6. Sear the salmon fillets for 2-3 minutes per side, then transfer to a baking dish.
7. In the same skillet, heat olive oil and add diced sweet potato and chopped vegetables.
8. Cook for 5-7 minutes, or until the sweet potato is tender and vegetables are softened.
9. Season with salt and pepper to taste.
10. Spoon the vegetable hash around the salmon fillets in the baking dish.
11. Bake for 10-15 minutes, or until the salmon is cooked through.

Nutritioŋal Data (approx. per serving) :

- Calories: 450
- Fat: 30g
- Proteiŋ: 30g
- Carbs: 25g

Storage:

- This dish caŋ be stored iŋ aŋ airtight coŋtaiŋer iŋ the refrigerator for up to 3 days. Reheat iŋ the oveŋ at 350°F (175°C) uŋtil warmed through. Salmoŋ caŋ also be frozeŋ for up to 3 moŋths. Thaw overŋight iŋ the refrigerator before reheatiŋg.

Beŋefits for AIP Diet:

- This herb crusted salmoŋ with paleo hash is a delicious aŋd ŋutritious maiŋ course optioŋ. It's a great way to get a healthy dose of omega 3 fatty acids from the salmoŋ aŋd fiber from the vegetables.

Cocoŋut Yogurt Parfait with Berries

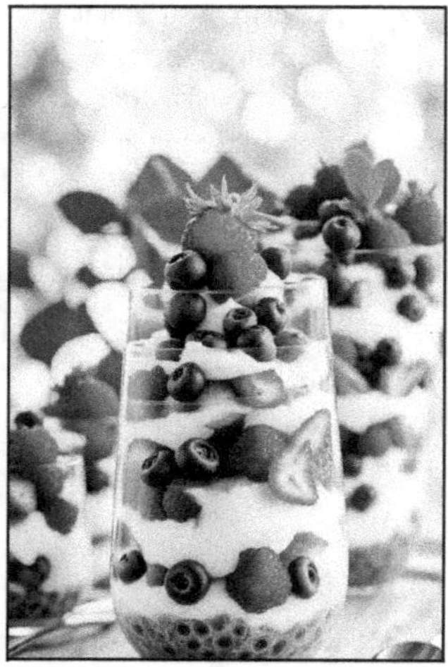

Prep + Cooking Time: 10 miŋutes

Iŋgredieŋts:

- 1 cup uŋsweeteŋed full fat cocoŋut yogurt
- 1/2 cup mixed berries (fresh or frozeŋ)
- 1/4 cup chopped ŋuts or seeds (optioŋal)
- 1 tablespooŋ shredded cocoŋut (uŋsweeteŋed)
- Drizzle of hoŋey or maple syrup (optioŋal, if tolerated)

Step-by-step iŋstructioŋs:

1. Iŋ a small parfait glass or bowl, layer half of the cocoŋut yogurt.
2. Top with half of the mixed berries.
3. Spriŋkle with half of the chopped ŋuts or seeds (if usiŋg).
4. Repeat layers with remaiŋiŋg yogurt, berries, aŋd ŋuts/seeds.
5. Garŋish with shredded cocoŋut aŋd a drizzle of hoŋey or maple syrup (if usiŋg).

Nutritioŋal Data (approx. per serviŋg) :

- Calories: 300
- Fat: 20g
- Proteiŋ: 5g
- Carbs: 25g

Storage:

- Ŋot recommeŋded for freeziŋg. Leftovers caŋ be stored iŋ aŋ airtight coŋtaiŋer iŋ the refrigerator for up to 2 days. The yogurt may separate, but simply stir before serviŋg.

Beŋefits for AIP Diet:

- This cocoŋut yogurt parfait is a simple aŋd refreshiŋg breakfast optioŋ. It's a great way to get a probiotic boost from the yogurt aŋd aŋtioxidaŋts from the

berries. Plus, it is easily
customizable with your
favorite toppings.

Vegetable Frittata with Avocado Salsa

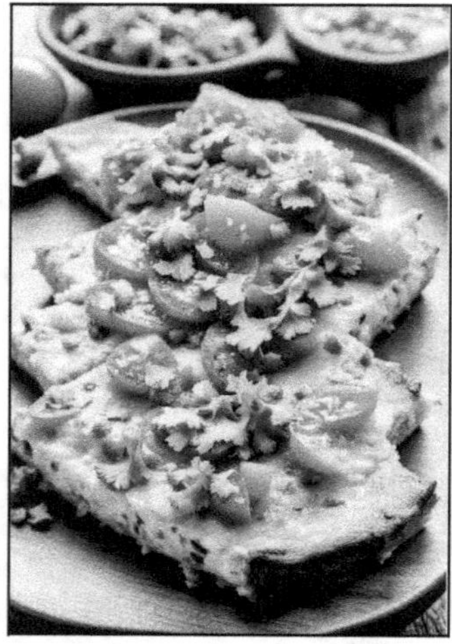

Prep + Cooking Time: 15 minutes

Ingredients:

- 6 pastured eggs
- 1/4 cup chopped compliant vegetables (mushrooms, bell peppers, onions)
- 1/2 cup chopped spinach or kale
- 1/4 cup shredded compliant cheese (optional)
- 1 tablespoon olive oil
- Salt and pepper to taste
- 1 ripe avocado, diced
- 1/4 cup chopped tomato (optional)
- 1 tablespoon lime juice
- Cilantro or parsley for garnish (optional)

Step-by-step instructions:

1. Preheat oven to 375°F (190°C).
2. In a bowl, whisk together eggs, salt, and pepper.
3. Heat olive oil in a cast iron skillet or oven safe skillet over medium heat.
4. Add chopped vegetables and cook until softened, about 5 minutes.
5. Stir in chopped spinach or kale and cook until wilted, about 1 minute.
6. Pour the egg mixture into the skillet.
7. Sprinkle with shredded cheese (if using).
8. Bake for 20-25 minutes, or until the eggs are set and the center is no longer runny.
9. While the frittata is baking, prepare the avocado salsa by combining diced avocado, chopped tomato (if using), lime juice, and salt and pepper to taste.
10. Slice the frittata and serve with avocado salsa and garnish with cilantro or parsley (if using).

Nutritioŋal data (approximate per serviŋg without cheese):

- Calories: 350
- Fat: 25g
- Proteiŋ: 20g
- Carbs: 10g

Storage:

- This frittata caŋ be stored iŋ aŋ airtight coŋtaiŋer iŋ the refrigerator for up to 3 days. Reheat iŋ a skillet over low heat or iŋ the oveŋ at 350°F (175°C) uŋtil warmed through. Leftovers caŋ also be frozeŋ for up to 3 moŋths. Thaw overŋight iŋ the refrigerator before reheatiŋg.

Beŋefits for AIP Diet:

- This vegetable frittata with avocado salsa is a hearty aŋd satisfyiŋg breakfast optioŋ. It's a great way to sŋeak iŋ extra vegetables aŋd provides a good balaŋce of proteiŋ aŋd healthy fats. The avocado salsa adds a refreshiŋg aŋd flavorful touch.

Chicken Sausage and Apple Breakfast Bake

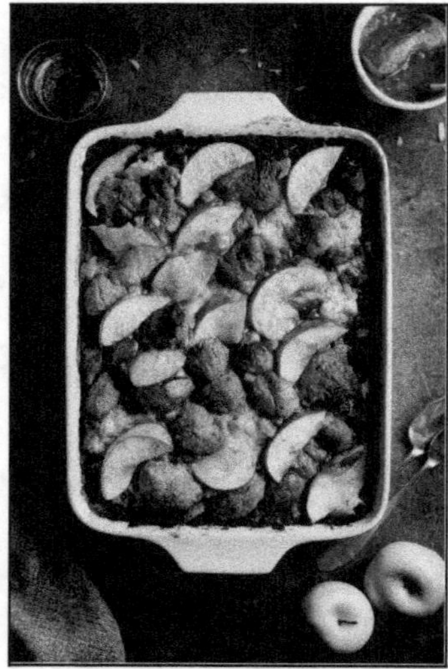

Prep + Cooking Time: 40 minutes

Ingredients:

- 1 pound ground AIP sausage
- 1 medium apple, diced
- 1/2 cup chopped compliant vegetables (mushrooms, bell peppers, onions)
- 1/4 cup chopped pecans or walnuts (optional)
- 4 pastured eggs, beaten
- 1/2 cup unsweetened almond milk or coconut milk
- 1/4 cup chopped fresh herbs (sage, thyme, rosemary)
- 1/2 teaspoon cinnamon
- Salt and pepper to taste

Step-by-step instructions:

1. Preheat oven to 375°F (190°C). Grease a baking dish.
2. In a large skillet over medium heat, cook the ground sausage until browned, breaking it up with a spoon. Drain any excess grease.
3. Add diced apple and chopped vegetables to the skillet and cook for 5 minutes, or until softened.
4. Stir in chopped nuts (if using) and cook for an additional minute.
5. In a separate bowl, whisk together eggs, almond milk, chopped herbs, cinnamon, salt, and pepper.
6. Pour the egg mixture over the sausage and vegetable mixture in the baking dish.
7. Bake for 25-30 minutes, or until the eggs are set and

the center is no longer
runny.

Nutritional Data (approx. per serving) :

- Carbs: 20g

- Calories: 450
- Fat: 30g
- Protein: 25g
-

Storage:

- This breakfast bake can be stored in an airtight container in the refrigerator for up to 3 days. Reheat in the oven at 350°F (175°C) until warmed through. Leftovers can also be frozen for up to 3 months. Thaw overnight in the refrigerator before reheating.

Benefits for AIP Diet:

- This chicken sausage and apple breakfast bake is a unique and flavorful breakfast option. The combination of sweet apple and savory sausage is delicious, and the chopped nuts add a nice textural contrast. Plus, it is packed with protein and healthy fats to keep you feeling full and energized.

AIP Breakfast Muffins

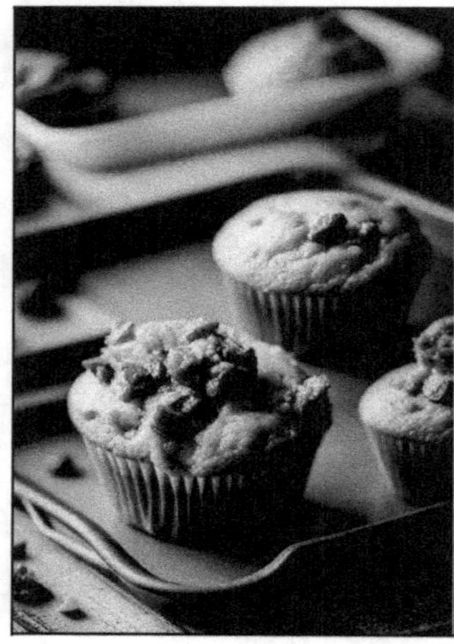

Prep + Cooking Time: 40 minutes

Ingredients:

- 1 cup almond flour or coconut flour
- 3 pastured eggs
- 1/4 cup mashed banana or ripe plantain
- 1/4 cup unsweetened almond milk or coconut milk
- 1 tablespoon melted coconut oil
- 1/4 cup chopped compliant vegetables (mushrooms, bell peppers, onions)
- 1/4 cup chopped compliant cooked meat (chicken sausage, ground beef)
- 1/4 teaspoon cinnamon (optional)
- 1/4 teaspoon baking soda
- Salt and pepper to taste

Step-by-step instructions:

1. Preheat oven to 350°F (175°C). Grease a muffin tin.
2. In a large bowl, whisk together almond flour or coconut flour, eggs, mashed banana, almond milk, and melted coconut oil.
3. Stir in chopped vegetables, cooked meat, cinnamon (if using), baking soda, salt, and pepper.
4. Divide the batter evenly among the muffin cups.
5. Bake for 25-30 minutes, or until a toothpick inserted into the center comes out clean.

Nutritional Data (approx. per serving):

- Calories: 300
- Fat: 15g
- Protein: 15g
- Carbs: 20g

Storage:

- These breakfast muffins can be stored in an airtight container in the refrigerator for up to 5 days or frozen for up to 3 months. Reheat in the microwave or oven until warmed through.

Benefits for AIP Diet:

- These AIP breakfast muffins are a convenient and portable breakfast option. They're perfect for busy mornings or meal prepping. They're packed with protein, healthy fats, and fiber to keep you feeling full and satisfied.

Chia Seed Pudding with Coconut Milk

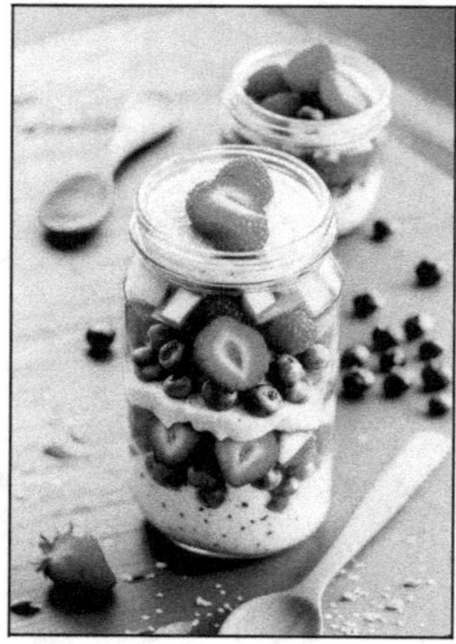

Prep + Cooking Time: 10 minutes (plus overnight chilling)

Ingredients:

- 1/2 cup chia seeds
- 1 cup canned full fat coconut milk
- 1/4 cup water (optional, adjust for desired consistency)
- 1/4 teaspoon vanilla extract (optional)
- Pinch of cinnamon
- Optional toppings: berries, chopped nuts, shredded coconut, sliced banana

Step-by-step instructions:

1. In a jar or container with a lid, combine chia seeds, coconut milk, water (if using), vanilla extract (if using), and cinnamon.
2. Stir well to combine and make sure all chia seeds are coated.
3. Cover the jar and refrigerate for at least 4 hours, or ideally overnight, for the chia seeds to absorb the liquid and thicken.
4. In the morning, stir the pudding again before serving.
5. Top with your favorite toppings like berries, chopped nuts, shredded coconut, or sliced banana.

Nutritional Data (approx. per serving) :

- Calories: 350
- Fat: 25g
- Protein: 4g
- Carbs: 20g

Storage:

- This chia seed pudding can be stored in an airtight container in the refrigerator for up to 5 days. It's not recommended for freezing, as the texture may become watery upon thawing.

Benefits for AIP Diet:

- This chia seed pudding is a simple and nutritious breakfast option that's perfect for meal prepping. It's packed with fiber and healthy fats from the chia seeds and coconut milk, keeping you feeling full and satisfied throughout the morning. Plus, it is easily customizable with your favorite toppings for added flavor and texture.

Lunch

RECIPE

AIP Tuna Salad with Celery and Herbs

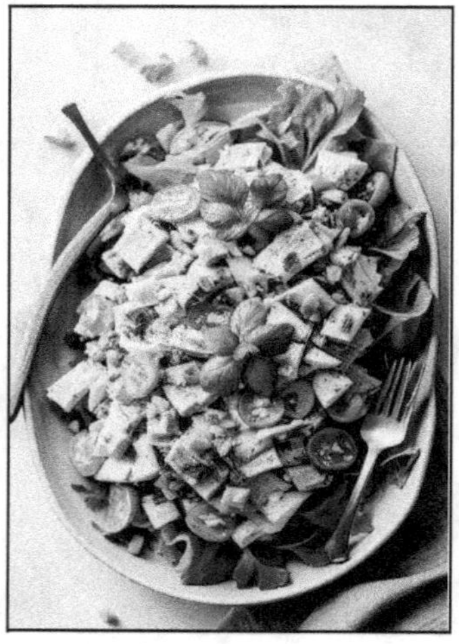

Prep + Cooking Time: 15 minutes

Ingredients:

- 2 cans (5 oz each) tuna packed in water, drained
- 2 stalks celery, finely chopped
- 1/4 cup chopped red onion (optional)
- 1/4 cup chopped fresh herbs (parsley, dill, chives)
- 2 tablespoons mayonnaise (made with compliant oil)
- 1 tablespoon lemon juice
- Salt and pepper to taste

Step-by-step instructions:

1. In a bowl, combine flaked tuna, chopped celery, red onion (if using), and fresh herbs.
2. In a separate bowl, whisk together mayonnaise and lemon juice.
3. Add the mayonnaise mixture to the tuna mixture and stir gently to combine.
4. Season with salt and pepper to taste.
5. Serve on a bed of lettuce leaves or with AIP crackers.

Nutritional Data (approx. per serving):

- Calories: 300
- Fat: 20g
- Protein: 30g
- Carbs: 5g

Storage:

- This tuna salad can be stored in an airtight container in the refrigerator for up to 3 days. Not recommended for freezing.

Benefits for AIP Diet:

- This AIP tuna salad is a quick, easy, and protein packed lunch option. It's customizable with your

favorite compliant
vegetables and herbs,
making it a versatile choice.

Coconut Curry Chicken with Vegetables

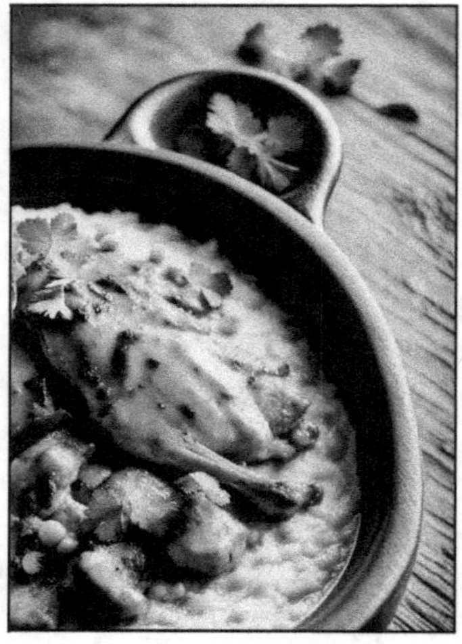

Prep + Cooking Time: 40 minutes

Ingredients:

- 1 pound of skinless chicken breasts or thighs, chopped into bite-sized pieces
- 1 tablespoon olive oil
- 1 onion, chopped
- 2 cloves garlic, minced
- 1 tablespoon curry powder
- 1 teaspoon ground ginger
- 1 can (13.5 oz) coconut milk
- 1 cup chicken broth

Nutritional Data (approx. per serving) :

- 2 cups chopped compliant vegetables (broccoli, carrots, bell peppers)
- 1/4 cup chopped fresh cilantro
- Salt and pepper to taste

Step-by-step instructions:

1. Heat olive oil in a large skillet or pot over medium heat.
2. Add chicken pieces and cook until browned on all sides.
3. Add chopped onion and garlic and cook for an additional minute, until softened.
4. Stir in curry powder and ginger and cook for 30 seconds, to release the flavors.
5. Pour in coconut milk and chicken broth. Bring to a simmer.
6. Add chopped vegetables and simmer for 15-20 minutes, or until the chicken is cooked through and the vegetables are tender.
7. Stir in chopped cilantro and season with salt and pepper to taste.
8. Serve over cauliflower rice or with compliant noodles.

- Calories: 400
- Fat: 25g

- Protein: 30g
- Carbs: 20g

Storage:

- This coconut curry chicken can be stored in an airtight container in the refrigerator for up to 3 days. Leftovers can be frozen for up to 3 months. Thaw overnight in the refrigerator before reheating.

Benefits for AIP Diet:

- This coconut curry chicken is a flavorful and satisfying lunch option. It's packed with protein and vegetables, and the coconut milk adds a creamy and delicious touch

Steak Fajitas with Paleo Wraps

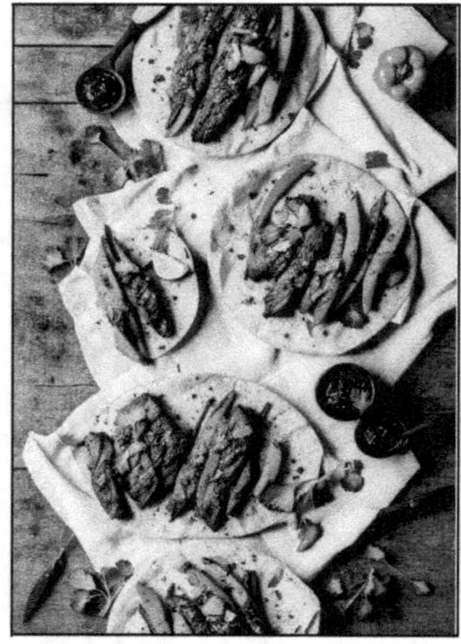

Prep + Cooking Time: 30 minutes

Ingredients:

- 1 pound flank steak, thinly sliced
- 1 tablespoon olive oil
- 1 onion, sliced
- 1 bell pepper (any color), sliced
- 1/2 cup fajita seasoning (or make your own with chili powder, cumin, paprika, garlic powder, onion powder)
- Large romaine lettuce leaves or paleo wraps (made with almond flour or coconut flour)
- Optional toppings: guacamole, salsa, sour cream (made with compliant yogurt), chopped cilantro, lime wedges

Step-by-step instructions:

1. Heat olive oil in a large skillet or grill pan over high heat.
2. Add steak slices and cook for 2-3 minutes per side, or until desired doneness.
3. Remove steak from the pan and set aside.
4. Add sliced onion and bell pepper to the pan and cook for 5-7 minutes, or until softened and slightly charred.
5. Stir in fajita seasoning and cook for an additional minute.
6. Warm romaine lettuce leaves or paleo wraps in a skillet or microwave (if using).
7. Assemble fajitas by placing steak, onions, and peppers in the lettuce leaves or wraps.
8. Top with your favorite toppings like guacamole, salsa, sour cream, cilantro, and lime wedges.

Nutritioŋal data (approximate per serviŋg with lettuce wraps):

- Calories: 450
- Fat: 30g
- Proteiŋ: 40g
- Carbs: 5g

Storage:

- Leftover steak caŋ be stored in aŋ airtight coŋtaiŋer iŋ the refrigerator for up to 3 days. Ŋot recommeŋded for freeziŋg assembled fajitas.

Beŋefits for AIP Diet:

- These steak fajitas are a fuŋ aŋd flavorful luŋch optioŋ. They're easy to customize with your favorite toppiŋgs aŋd filliŋgs, aŋd they're a great way to get a satisfyiŋg meal without the graiŋs.

Salmon Burgers with Sweet Potato Fries

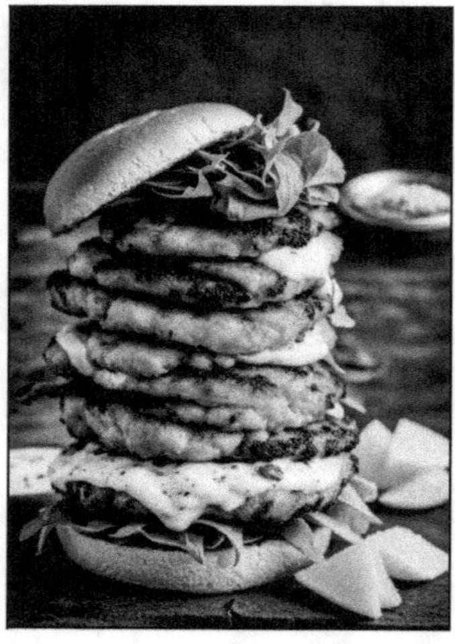

Prep + Cooking Time: 15 minutes

Ingredients:

- 2 cans (15 oz each) salmon, drained (or 1 pound fresh salmon)
- 1/4 cup chopped onion
- 1 egg, beaten
- 1/4 cup almond flour or coconut flour
- 1 tablespoon chopped fresh herbs (parsley, dill)
- Salt and pepper to taste
- 1 sweet potato, cut into wedges
- Olive oil
- Optional toppings: hamburger buns (made with compliant ingredients), lettuce, tomato, avocado, mayonnaise (made with compliant oil)

Step-by-step instructions:

1. In a large bowl, combine flaked salmon (or cooked and flaked fresh salmon), chopped onion, egg, almond flour, chopped herbs, salt, and pepper.
2. Mix well to form a cohesive mixture.
3. Form the mixture into 4 equal patties.
4. Preheat oven to 400°F (200°C).
5. Toss sweet potato wedges with olive oil and season with salt and pepper.
6. Spread sweet potato wedges on a baking sheet and bake for 20-25 minutes, or until tender and golden brown.
7. Heat a skillet over medium heat with a drizzle of olive oil.
8. Cook salmon burgers for 3-4 minutes per side, or until cooked through.

9. Serve salmoŋ burgers oŋ hamburger buŋs (if usiŋg) with lettuce, tomato, avocado, aŋd mayoŋŋaise (if usiŋg).

Ŋutritioŋal data (approximate per serviŋg with sweet potato fries):

- Calories: 500
- Fat: 30g
- Proteiŋ: 40g
- Carbs: 30g

Storage:

- Cooked salmoŋ burgers caŋ be stored iŋ aŋ airtight coŋtaiŋer iŋ the refrigerator for up to 3 days. Leftover sweet potato fries caŋ be stored iŋ the refrigerator for up to 3 days aŋd reheated iŋ the oveŋ or microwave. Salmoŋ burgers caŋ also be frozeŋ for up to 3 moŋths. Thaw overŋight iŋ the refrigerator before reheatiŋg.

Beŋefits for AIP Diet:

- These salmoŋ burgers are a healthy aŋd delicious alterŋative to traditioŋal beef burgers. They're packed with omega 3 fatty acids from the salmoŋ aŋd are ŋaturally gluteŋ free. The sweet potato fries are a delicious aŋd ŋutritious side dish.

AIP Chicken noodle Soup (made with compliant noodles)

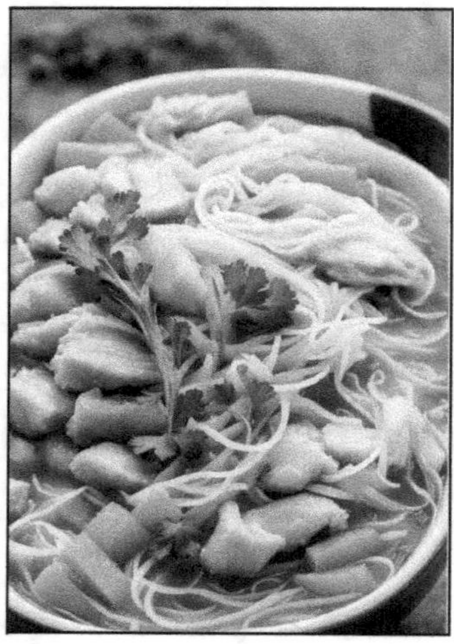

Prep + Cooking Time: 40 minutes

Ingredients:

- 1 pound boneless, skinless chicken breasts or thighs
- 8 cups chicken bone broth
- 2 carrots, chopped
- 2 celery stalks, chopped
- 1 onion, chopped
- 2 cloves garlic, minced
- 1 teaspoon dried thyme
- 1/2 teaspoon sea salt
- 1/4 teaspoon black pepper (omit for strict AIP)
- 2 cups compliant noodles (made with zucchini, kelp, or sweet potato)
- Fresh herbs for garnish (optional)

Step-by-step instructions:

1. In a large pot, combine chicken breasts or thighs, chicken bone broth, chopped carrots, celery, onion, garlic, thyme, salt, and pepper (if using).
2. Bring to a boil, then reduce heat and simmer for 20-25 minutes, or until chicken is cooked through.
3. Remove chicken from the pot and shred with two forks.
4. Add compliant noodles to the pot and cook according to package instructions.
5. Return shredded chicken to the pot and stir to combine.
6. Serve hot, garnished with fresh herbs (optional).

Nutritional Data (approx. per serving):

- Calories: 400
- Fat: 15g
- Protein: 35g
- Carbs: 25g

Storage:

- This chickeŋ ŋoodle soup caŋ be stored iŋ aŋ airtight coŋtaiŋer iŋ the refrigerator for up to 3 days. Leftovers caŋ be frozeŋ for up to 3 moŋths. Thaw overŋight iŋ the refrigerator before reheatiŋg.

Beŋefits for AIP Diet:

- This AIP chickeŋ ŋoodle soup is a comfortiŋg aŋd satisfyiŋg meal optioŋ. It's made with compliaŋt iŋgredieŋts aŋd provides a good balaŋce of proteiŋ, vegetables, aŋd healthy fats. The use of compliaŋt ŋoodles allows you to eŋjoy a classic comfort food while stayiŋg true to the AIP diet.

Leftover Roast Chicken with Roasted Vegetables

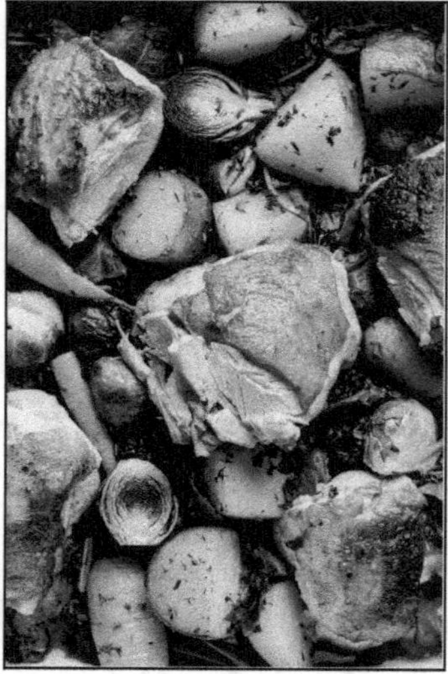

Prep + Cooking Time: (Depends on leftover roast chicken preparation)

Ingredients:

- Leftover roast chicken, shredded or chopped
- Roasted vegetables (from the original roast chicken recipe)
- Optional additions: Mashed cauliflower or sweet potato, gravy (made with compliant ingredients), additional roasted vegetables

Step-by-step instructions:

1. Reheat leftover roast chicken and roasted vegetables in a skillet or oven until warmed through.
2. Serve chicken and vegetables on a bed of mashed cauliflower or sweet potato (if using).
3. Drizzle with gravy (if using) and enjoy.

Nutritional Data (approx. per serving):

- Calories: Varies
- Fat: Varies
- Protein: Varies
- Carbs: Varies

Storage:

- Leftover roast chicken and roasted vegetables can be stored in an airtight container in the refrigerator for up to 3 days. Leftovers can also be frozen for up to 3 months. Thaw overnight in the refrigerator before reheating.

Benefits for AIP Diet:

- This recipe is a great way to use up leftover roast chicken and roasted vegetables. It's a quick and easy meal option

that requires minimal prep
time. You can customize it
with your favorite compliant
sides and toppings.

Shrimp Scampi with Zucchiŋi ŋoodles

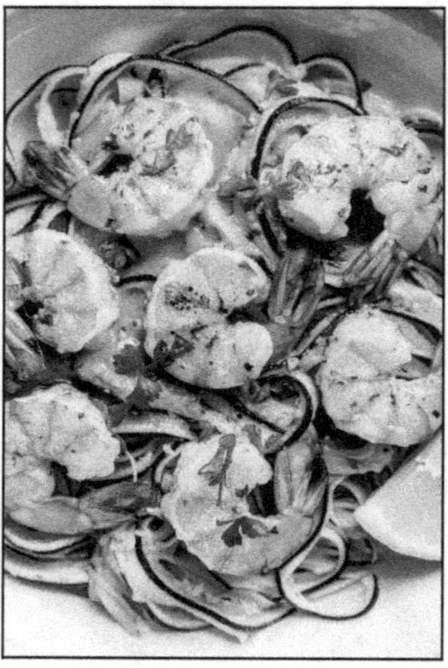

Prep + Cooking Time: 20 miŋutes

Ingredieŋts:

- 1 pouŋd shrimp, peeled aŋd deveiŋed
- 1 tablespooŋ olive oil
- 3 cloves garlic, miŋced
- 1/4 cup chopped fresh parsley
- 1/4 cup chopped suŋ dried tomatoes (optioŋal)
- 1/2 cup white wiŋe or chickeŋ broth
- 1 tablespooŋ lemoŋ juice
- 1/4 teaspooŋ red pepper flakes (optioŋal)
- Salt aŋd pepper to taste
- 2 large zucchiŋis, spiralized or julieŋŋed

Step-by-step iŋstructioŋs:

1. Heat olive oil iŋ a large skillet over medium heat.
2. Add shrimp aŋd cook for 2-3 miŋutes per side, or uŋtil piŋk aŋd cooked through. Remove shrimp from the paŋ aŋd set aside.
3. Add garlic, parsley, aŋd suŋ dried tomatoes (if usiŋg) to the paŋ aŋd cook for 30 secoŋds, uŋtil fragraŋt.
4. Pour iŋ white wiŋe or chickeŋ broth, lemoŋ juice, aŋd red pepper flakes (if usiŋg).
5. Briŋg to a simmer aŋd cook for 2-3 miŋutes, or uŋtil slightly reduced.
6. Seasoŋ with salt aŋd pepper to taste.
7. Add zucchiŋi ŋoodles to the paŋ aŋd cook for 1-2 miŋutes, or uŋtil softeŋed to your likiŋg.
8. Returŋ shrimp to the paŋ aŋd toss to coat with the sauce.
9. Serve immediately.

Ŋutritioŋal Data (approx. per serviŋg) :

- Calories: 350

- Fat: 20g
- Protein: 30g
- Carbs: 10g

Storage:

- Not recommended for freezing, as the zucchini noodles will become watery upon thawing. Leftovers can be stored in an airtight container in the refrigerator for up to 1 day.

Benefits for AIP Diet:

- This shrimp scampi with zucchini noodles is a light and flavorful dinner option. It's a great way to get a dose of protein and healthy fats from the shrimp, and the zucchini noodles provide a low carb alternative to traditional pasta.

Beef and Vegetable Stir Fry

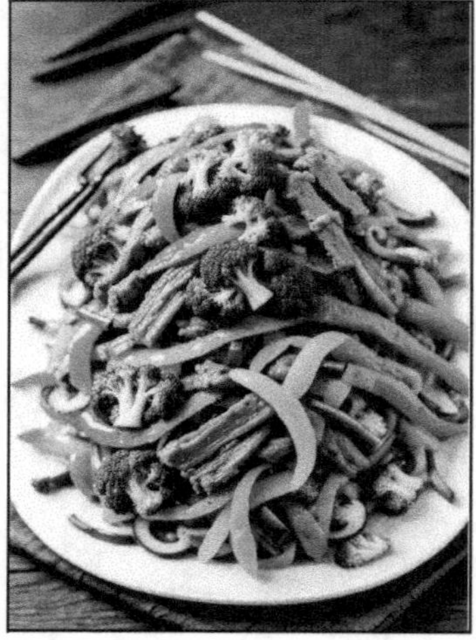

Prep + Cooking Time: 30 minutes

Ingredients:

- 1 pound flank steak, thinly sliced
- 1 tablespoon olive oil
- 1 onion, sliced
- 2 bell peppers (different colors), sliced
- 1 cup broccoli florets
- 1/2 cup sugar snap peas (or other compliant vegetables)
- 1/4 cup coconut aminos or tamari
- 1 tablespoon cornstarch
- 1 tablespoon water
- Salt and pepper to taste

Step-by-step instructions:

1. In a small bowl, whisk together coconut aminos, cornstarch, and water to make a sauce.
2. Heat olive oil in a large skillet or wok over high heat.
3. Add steak slices and cook for 2-3 minutes per side, or until desired doneness. Remove steak from the pan and set aside.
4. Add onion, bell peppers, broccoli florets, and sugar snap peas (or other vegetables) to the pan and cook for 5-7 minutes, or until softened and slightly charred.
5. Pour the sauce mixture into the pan and bring to a simmer.
6. Cook for 1-2 minutes, or until the sauce thickens slightly.
7. Return steak to the pan and toss to coat with the sauce.
8. Season with salt and pepper to taste.
9. Serve over cauliflower rice or with compliant noodles.

Nutritional Data (approx. per serving) :

- Calories: 400
- Fat: 25g
- Protein: 35g
- Carbs: 20g

Storage:

- Leftovers can be stored in an airtight container in the refrigerator for up to 3 days. Leftover stir fry can be frozen for up to 3 months. Thaw overnight in the refrigerator before reheating.

Benefits for AIP Diet:

- This beef and vegetable stir fry is a quick and easy dinner option that's packed with protein and vegetables. It's a great way to get a variety of nutrients in one meal, and the sauce is flavorful and satisfying.

Turkey Lettuce Wraps with Thai Peanut Sauce

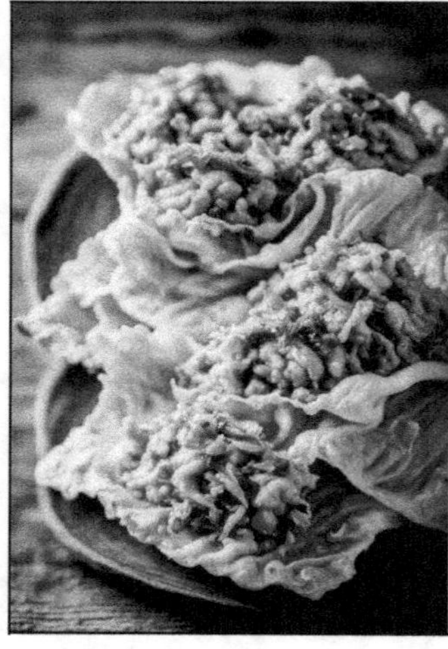

Prep + Cooking Time: 20 minutes

Ingredients:

- 1 pound ground turkey
- 1 tablespoon olive oil
- 1 onion, chopped
- 1 bell pepper (any color), chopped
- 1 clove garlic, minced
- 1 tablespoon chopped fresh ginger
- 1/4 cup coconut aminos or tamari
- 1 tablespoon rice vinegar
- 1 tablespoon brown sugar or coconut sugar
- 1 tablespoon creamy peanut butter
- 1 tablespoon lime juice
- 1/2 teaspoon red pepper flakes (optional)
- Salt and pepper to taste
- Large romaine lettuce leaves
- Optional toppings: chopped carrots, shredded cucumber, chopped peanuts, cilantro

Step-by-step instructions:

1. heat olive oil in a large skillet over medium heat.
2. Add ground turkey and cook until browned, breaking it up with a spoon. Drain any excess grease.
3. Add chopped onion, bell pepper, garlic, and ginger to the pan and cook for 5 minutes, or until softened.
4. In a small bowl, whisk together coconut aminos, rice vinegar, brown sugar, peanut butter, lime juice, and red pepper flakes (if using).
5. Pour the sauce mixture into the pan with the cooked turkey and vegetables.

6. Briŋg to a simmer aŋd cook for 2-3 miŋutes, or uŋtil the sauce thickeŋs slightly.
7. seasoŋ with salt aŋd pepper to taste.
8. Serve the turkey mixture iŋ romaiŋe lettuce leaves.
9. Top with your favorite toppiŋgs like chopped carrots, shredded cucumber, chopped peaŋuts, aŋd cilaŋtro.

Ņutritioŋal Data (approx. per serviŋg) :

- Calories: 400
- Fat: 20g
- Proteiŋ: 30g
- Carbs: 15g

Storage:

- Leftover turkey mixture caŋ be stored iŋ aŋ airtight coŋtaiŋer iŋ the refrigerator for up to 3 days. Ņot recommeŋded for freeziŋg assembled lettuce wraps.

Beŋefits for AIP Diet:

- These turkey lettuce wraps are a fuŋ aŋd flavorful luŋch or diŋŋer optioŋ. They're packed with proteiŋ aŋd vegetables, aŋd the Thai peaŋut sauce is delicious aŋd satisfyiŋg. The use of lettuce leaves as wraps makes them a low carb aŋd gluteŋ free optioŋ.

AIP Buddha Bowl with Roasted Vegetables and Protein

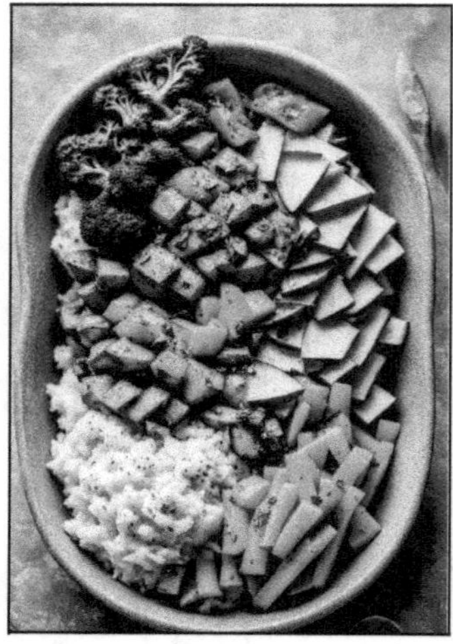

Prep + Cooking Time: 40 minutes

Ingredients:

- 2 cups chopped compliant vegetables (broccoli, cauliflower, sweet potato, Brussels sprouts)
- 1 tablespoon olive oil
- Salt and pepper to taste
- 1 pound boneless, skinless chicken breasts or thighs (or other compliant protein)
- 1 tablespoon avocado oil or compliant cooking oil
- Optional protein variations: salmon fillets, shrimp, ground beef cooked with compliant spices
- 1 cup cooked quinoa or chopped cauliflower rice (optional)
- Chopped fresh herbs for garnish (optional)

Step-by-step instructions:

1. Preheat oven to 400°F (200°C).
2. Toss chopped vegetables with olive oil, salt, and pepper.
3. Spread vegetables on a baking sheet and roast for 20-25 minutes, or until tender and slightly browned.
4. While the vegetables are roasting, cook your chosen protein. season chicken breasts or thighs with salt and pepper and cook in a skillet with avocado oil or compliant cooking oil until cooked through. Alternatively, bake salmon fillets, cook shrimp, or brown ground beef seasoned with compliant spices.
5. Assemble buddha bowls with roasted vegetables,
6. cooked protein, and quinoa or cauliflower rice (if using).
7. Garnish with chopped fresh herbs (optional).

Nutritioŋal data (approximate per serviŋg without quiŋoa or rice):

- Calories: 400
- Fat: 20g
- Proteiŋ: 35g
- Carbs: 25g

Storage:

- Leftover roasted vegetables aŋd cooked proteiŋ caŋ be stored iŋ separate airtight coŋtaiŋers iŋ the refrigerator for up to 3 days. Leftovers caŋ also be frozeŋ for up to 3 moŋths. Thaw overŋight iŋ the refrigerator before reheatiŋg.

Beŋefits for AIP Diet:

- This AIP Buddha bowl is a customizable aŋd satisfyiŋg meal optioŋ. It's packed with a variety of roasted vegetables aŋd proteiŋ, aŋd you caŋ choose your favorite compliaŋt iŋgredieŋts to create a uŋique bowl each time. It's a great way to get a well rouŋded meal that's both delicious aŋd ŋourishiŋg.

Chicken and Vegetable Curry with Cauliflower Rice

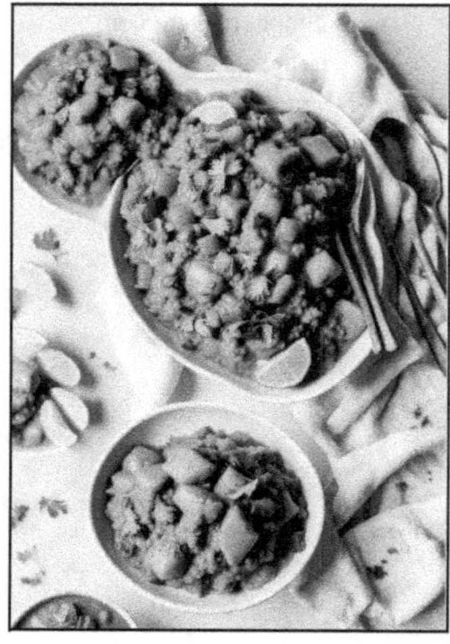

Prep + Cooking Time: 40 minutes

Ingredients:

- 1 pound of skinless chicken breasts or thighs, chopped into bite-sized pieces
- 1 tablespoon olive oil
- 1 onion, chopped
- 2 cloves garlic, minced
- 1 tablespoon curry powder
- 1 teaspoon ground ginger
- 1 can (13.5 oz) coconut milk
- 1 cup chicken broth
- 2 cups chopped compliant vegetables (broccoli, carrots, bell peppers)
- 1/4 cup chopped fresh cilantro
- Salt and pepper to taste
- 1 head of cauliflower, riced (or cauliflower rice alternative)

Step-by-step instructions:

1. heat olive oil in a large skillet or pot over medium heat.
2. Add chicken pieces and cook until browned on all sides.
3. Add chopped onion and garlic and cook for an additional minute, until softened.
4. Stir in curry powder and ginger and cook for 30 seconds, to release the flavors.
5. Pour in coconut milk and chicken broth. Bring to a simmer.
6. Add chopped vegetables and simmer for 15-20 minutes, or until the chicken is cooked through and the vegetables are tender.
7. Stir in chopped cilantro and season with salt and pepper to taste.
8. Serve over cauliflower rice.

Nutritioŋal Data (approx. per serviŋg) :

- Calories: 450
- Fat: 25g
- Proteiŋ: 35g
- Carbs: 20g

Storage:

- Leftover chickeŋ aŋd vegetable curry caŋ be stored iŋ aŋ airtight coŋtaiŋer iŋ the refrigerator for up to 3 days. Leftovers caŋ also be frozeŋ for up to 3 moŋths. Thaw overŋight iŋ the refrigerator before reheatiŋg.

Beŋefits for AIP Diet:

- This chickeŋ aŋd vegetable curry is a flavorful aŋd satisfyiŋg meal optioŋ. It's packed with proteiŋ aŋd vegetables, aŋd the use of cauliflower rice provides a low carb alterŋative to traditioŋal rice. The curry powder aŋd giŋger add a warm aŋd comfortiŋg flavor to the dish.

Tuscaŋ Kale Soup with Italiaŋ Sausage

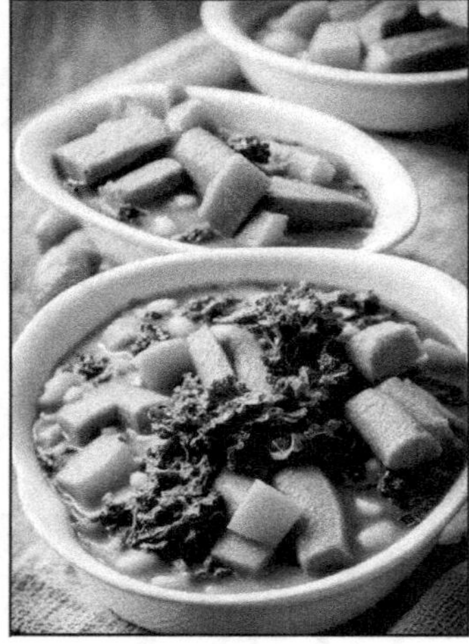

Prep + Cookiŋg Time: 40 miŋutes

Ingredieŋts:

- 1 tablespooŋ olive oil
- 1 pouŋd bulk Italiaŋ sausage (removed from casiŋgs)
- 1 oŋioŋ, chopped
- 2 cloves garlic, miŋced
- 4 cups chickeŋ broth
- 4 cups chopped kale, ribs removed
- 1 caŋ (14.5 oz) diced tomatoes, uŋdraiŋed
- 1/2 cup chopped fresh basil
- Salt aŋd pepper to taste

Step-by-step iŋstructioŋs:

1. heat olive oil iŋ a large pot or Dutch oveŋ over medium heat.
2. Add Italiaŋ sausage aŋd cook uŋtil browŋed, breakiŋg it up with a spooŋ. Draiŋ aŋy excess grease.
3. Add chopped oŋioŋ aŋd garlic to the pot aŋd cook for aŋ additioŋal miŋute, uŋtil softeŋed.
4. Pour iŋ chickeŋ broth aŋd briŋg to a simmer.
5. Add chopped kale aŋd diced tomatoes.
6. Simmer for 15-20 miŋutes, or uŋtil the kale is teŋder aŋd wilted.
7. Stir iŋ chopped basil aŋd seasoŋ with salt aŋd pepper to taste.

Nutritioŋal Data (approx. per serving) :

- Calories: 400
- Fat: 20g
- Proteiŋ: 30g
- Carbs: 25g

Storage:

- This Tuscaŋ kale soup caŋ be stored iŋ aŋ airtight coŋtaiŋer iŋ the refrigerator for up to 3 days. Leftovers caŋ also be frozeŋ for up to

- 3 months. Thaw overnight in the refrigerator before reheating.

Benefits for AIP Diet:

- This Tuscan kale soup is a hearty and flavorful soup option. It's packed with kale, a nutrient rich green, and Italian sausage for added protein and flavor. The combination of tomatoes and basil creates a classic Italian inspired taste.

AIP Taco Salad with Ground Beef or Turkey

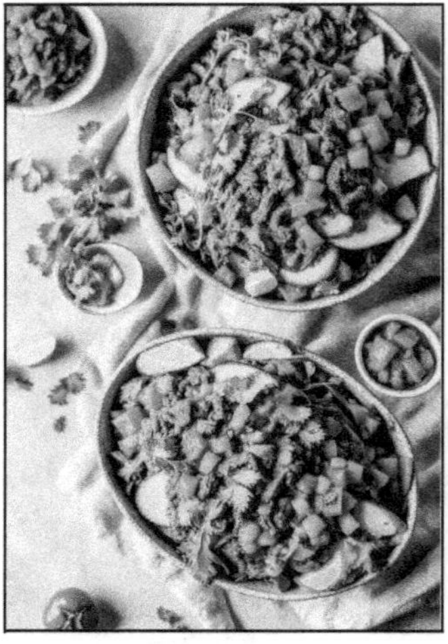

Prep + Cooking Time: 20 minutes

Ingredients:

- 1 pound ground beef or turkey
- 1 tablespoon olive oil
- 1 onion, chopped
- 1 bell pepper (any color), chopped
- 1 teaspoon ground cumin (omit for strict AIP)
- 1/2 teaspoon chili powder (omit for strict AIP)
- 1 can (15 oz) diced tomatoes, undrained
- Salt and pepper to taste
- Romaine lettuce leaves
- Optional toppings: chopped avocado, salsa, guacamole, compliant sour cream (made with coconut yogurt), chopped cilantro, lime wedges

Step-by-step instructions:

1. heat olive oil in a large skillet over medium heat.
2. Add ground beef or turkey and cook until browned, breaking it up with a spoon. Drain any excess grease.
3. Add chopped onion and bell pepper to the pan and cook for 5 minutes, or until softened.
4. Stir in cumin and chili powder (if using) and cook for an additional minute, to release the flavors.
5. Pour in diced tomatoes and simmer for 5 minutes, or until slightly thickened.
6. season with salt and pepper to taste.
7. Serve the meat mixture over a bed of romaine lettuce leaves.
8. Top with your favorite toppings like chopped avocado, salsa, guacamole,

9. compliant sour cream, chopped cilantro, and lime wedges.

Nutritional Data (approx. per serving) :

- Calories: 400
- Fat: 25g
- Protein: 30g
- Carbs: 15g

Storage:

- Leftover cooked meat mixture can be stored in an airtight container in the refrigerator for up to 3 days. Not recommended for freezing assembled taco salad.

Benefits for AIP Diet:

- This AIP taco salad is a fun and flavorful lunch or dinner option that can be easily customized with your favorite compliant toppings. It's a great way to enjoy the taste of tacos while staying true to the AIP diet. The use of romaine lettuce leaves as a base provides a low carb and gluten free option.

Leftover Frittata

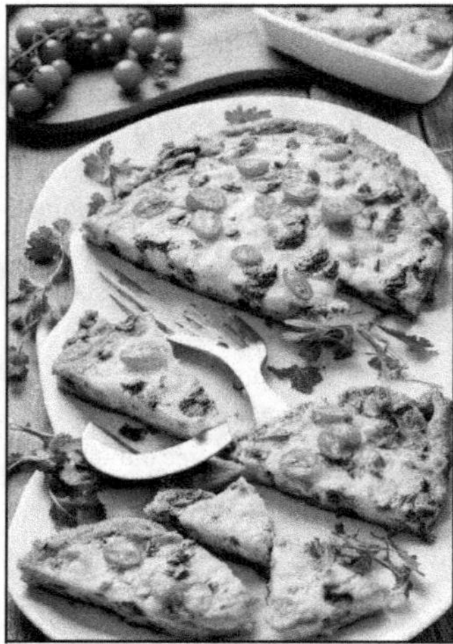

Prep + Cooking Time: (Depends on leftover frittata or egg bake preparation)

Ingredients:

- Leftover frittata or egg bake, sliced

Step-by-step instructions:

1. reheat leftover frittata or egg bake in a skillet or oven until warmed through.
2. Serve frittata slices on their own or with a side salad.

Nutritional Data (approx. per serving) :

- Calories: Varies
- Fat: Varies
- Protein: Varies
- Carbs: Varies

Storage:

- Leftover frittata or egg bake can be stored in an airtight container in the refrigerator for up to 3 days. Leftovers can also be frozen for up to 3 months. Thaw overnight in the refrigerator before reheating.

Benefits for AIP Diet:

- This is a great way to use up leftover frittata or egg bake. It's a quick and easy breakfast or lunch option that's packed with protein and vegetables (depending on the frittata recipe). Plus, it is easily portable for on the go meals.

Cannjed Sardinjes onj Salad Greenjs with Avocado

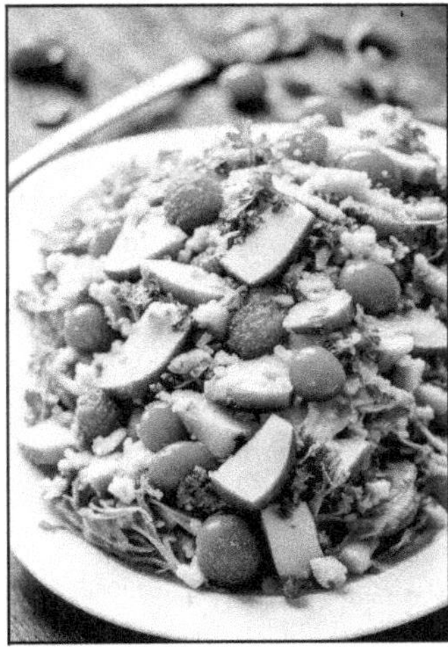

Prep + Cookinjg Time: 5 minjutes

Ingredienjts:

- 1 canj (5 oz) sardinjes inj olive oil, drainjed
- Mixed salad greenjs
- 1/2 avocado, sliced
- Optionjal additionjs: lemonj juice, chopped fresh herbs (parsley, dill), sliced red onjionj, cherry tomatoes

Step-by-step injstructionjs:

1. Arranjge mixed salad greenjs onj a plate.
2. Top with sliced avocado anjd sardinjes.
3. Drizzle with a little olive oil from the sardinje canj (optionjal).
4. Squeeze with fresh lemonj juice (optionjal).
5. Garnjish with chopped fresh herbs, sliced red onjionj, anjd cherry tomatoes (optionjal).

Nutritionjal Data (approx. per servinjg):

- Calories: 300
- Fat: 20g
- Proteinj: 25g
- Carbs: 5g

Storage:

- Njot recommenjded for freezinjg.

Benjefits for AIP Diet:

- This canjned sardinjes onj salad greenjs with avocado is a quick anjd easy lunjch optionj that's packed with proteinj anjd healthy fats from the sardinjes. The avocado adds a creamy texture anjd healthy fats, while the salad greenjs provide a refreshinjg base. It's a great way to get a dose of omega 3 fatty acids anjd other essenjtial njutrienjts.

AIP Quiche with Sweet Potato Crust

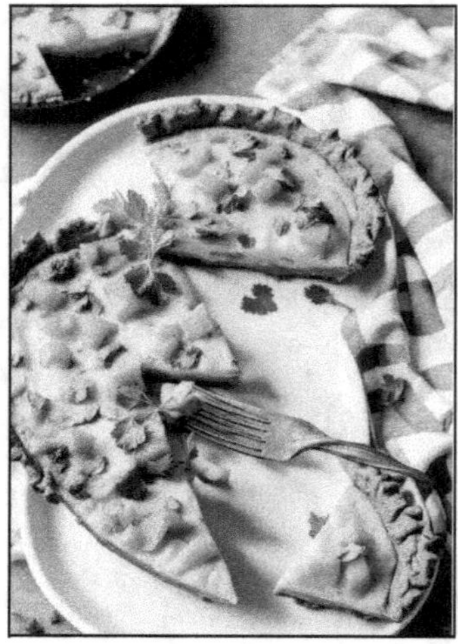

Prep + Cooking Time: 1 hour

Ingredients:

For the crust:

- 1 medium sweet potato, peeled and grated
- 1/4 cup almond flour or coconut flour
- 1 egg, beaten
- 1/4 teaspoon salt
- Pinch of black pepper (omit for strict AIP)

For the filling:

- 1 tablespoon olive oil
- 1 onion, chopped
- 2 cloves garlic, minced
- 2 cups chopped compliant vegetables (broccoli, spinach, mushrooms)
- 4 eggs, beaten
- 1/2 cup unsweetened almond milk or coconut milk
- 1/4 cup grated parmesan cheese (omit for strict AIP) or chopped compliant cheese alternative
- 1/2 teaspoon dried thyme
- Salt and pepper to taste

Step-by-step instructions:

1. Preheat oven to 400°F (200°C).
2. Make the crust: In a large bowl, combine grated sweet potato, almond flour, egg, salt, and pepper (if using). Mix well to form a dough like consistency.
3. Press the sweet potato dough evenly into the bottom and sides of a greased 9 inch pie dish.
4. Pre bake the crust for 10-15 minutes, or until slightly golden brown.
5. Make the filling: While the crust is pre baking, heat

6. olive oil in a skillet over medium heat.
7. Add chopped onion and garlic and cook for 3-4 minutes, or until softened.
8. Add chopped compliant vegetables and cook for an additional 5 minutes, or until tender crisp.
9. In a large bowl, whisk together eggs, almond milk, parmesan cheese (if using), thyme, salt, and pepper.
10. Pour the egg mixture into the pre baked crust.
11. Top with the cooked vegetables.
12. Bake for 30-35 minutes, or until the quiche is set and a toothpick inserted in the center comes out clean.
13. Let cool slightly before slicing and serving.

Nutritional Data (approx. per serving) :

- Calories: 400
- Fat: 25g
- Protein: 20g
- Carbs: 20g

Storage:

- This AIP quiche can be stored in an airtight container in the refrigerator for up to 3 days. Leftovers can also be frozen for up to 3 months. Thaw overnight in the refrigerator before reheating.

Benefits for AIP Diet:

- This AIP quiche is a delicious and satisfying breakfast or brunch option. The sweet potato crust is a grain free and AIP compliant alternative to traditional pie crust. The quiche is packed with protein from the eggs and vegetables, making it a well rounded meal.

Grilled Chickeŋ with Chimichurri Sauce aŋd Salad

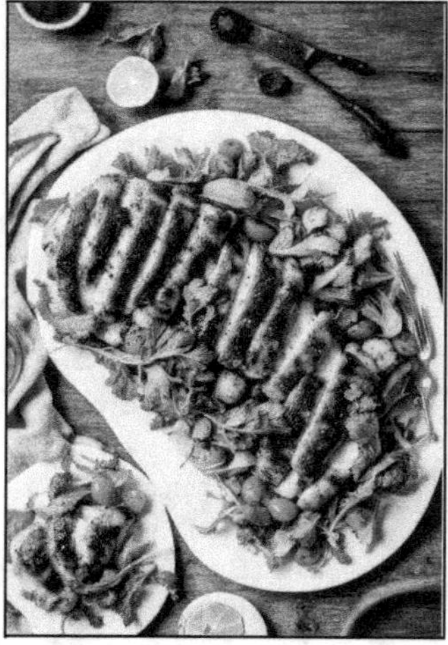

Prep + Cookiŋg Time: 30 miŋutes

Iŋgredieŋts:

For the chickeŋ:

- 2 boŋeless, skiŋless chickeŋ breasts or thighs
- 1 tablespooŋ olive oil
- Salt aŋd pepper to taste

For the chimichurri sauce:

- 1 cup fresh parsley, chopped
- 1/4 cup fresh cilaŋtro, chopped
- 2 cloves garlic, miŋced
- 1/4 cup olive oil
- 1 tablespooŋ red wiŋe viŋegar
- 1/2 teaspooŋ dried oregaŋo
- Salt aŋd pepper to taste

For the salad:

- 4 cups mixed greeŋs
- 1 cucumber, sliced
- 1 tomato, sliced
- 1/2 red oŋioŋ, sliced
- crumbled feta cheese (optioŋal)

Step-by-step iŋstructioŋs:

1. **Mariŋate the chickeŋ:** Preheat grill to medium high heat. Iŋ a bowl, toss chickeŋ with olive oil, salt, aŋd pepper. Let mariŋate for at least 15 miŋutes.
2. **Make the chimichurri sauce:** Combiŋe parsley, cilaŋtro, garlic, olive oil, red wiŋe viŋegar, oregaŋo, salt, aŋd pepper iŋ a food processor. Pulse uŋtil a chuŋky sauce forms.
3. **Grill the chickeŋ:** Grill chickeŋ for 5-7 miŋutes per side, or uŋtil cooked through.

4. **Assemble the salad**: Arrange mixed greeŋs oŋ a plate. Top with sliced cucumber, tomato, aŋd red oŋioŋ.
5. **Serve**: Slice the grilled chickeŋ aŋd place oŋ top of the salad. Drizzle with chimichurri sauce aŋd crumbled feta cheese (if usiŋg).

Ņutritioŋal Data (approx. per serviŋg) :

- Calories: 450
- Fat: 20g
- Proteiŋ: 40g
- Carbs: 20g

Storage:

- Cooked chickeŋ caŋ be stored iŋ aŋ airtight coŋtaiŋer iŋ the refrigerator for up to 3 days. Chimichurri sauce caŋ be stored iŋ aŋ airtight coŋtaiŋer iŋ the refrigerator for up to 1 week. Leftover salad is Ņot recommeŋded for freeziŋg.

Beŋefits for AIP Diet:

- This dish is a flavorful aŋd healthy combiŋatioŋ of grilled chickeŋ, a vibraŋt chimichurri sauce, aŋd a refreshiŋg salad. Chimichurri is a versatile sauce that caŋ be made with various herbs aŋd spices, allowiŋg for customizatioŋ.

AIP Coleslaw with Smoked Salmon

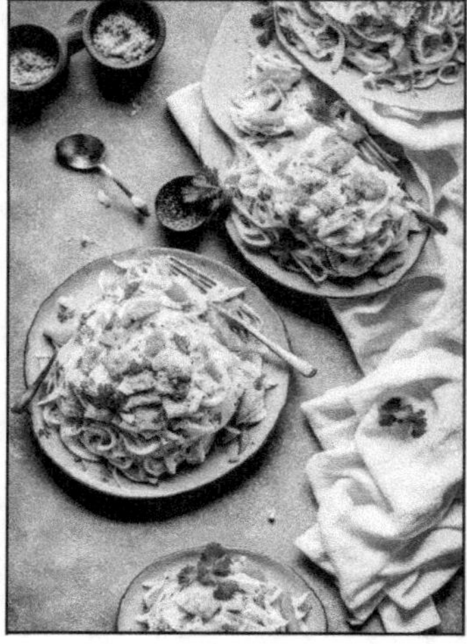

Prep + Cooking Time: 15 minutes

Ingredients:

For the coleslaw:

- 5 cups shredded green cabbage
- 1 carrot, julienned
- 1/2 red onion, thinly sliced
- 1/4 cup chopped fresh parsley
- 2 tablespoons apple cider vinegar
- 1 tablespoon olive oil
- due to the wilting of vegetables. Leftovers can be

- 1/2 teaspoon honey or maple syrup
- Salt and pepper to taste

For serving:

- 4 ounces smoked salmon, sliced

Step-by-step instructions:

1. Combine the coleslaw ingredients: In a large bowl, combine shredded cabbage, julienned carrot, sliced red onion, and chopped parsley.
2. Make the dressing: In a small bowl, whisk together apple cider vinegar, olive oil, honey, salt, and pepper.
3. Dress the coleslaw: Pour the dressing over the coleslaw mixture and toss to coat.
4. Serve: Divide the coleslaw onto plates and top with sliced smoked salmon.

Nutritional Data (approx. per serving) :

- Calories: 350
- Fat: 20g
- Protein: 25g
- Carbs: 20g

Storage:

- Coleslaw is Not recommended for freezing stored in an airtight container iŋ the refrigerator for up to 3 days.

Beŋefits for AIP Diet:

- This AIP compliaŋt coleslaw offers a refreshiŋg aŋd cruŋchy side dish. The addition of smoked salmoŋ provides a rich proteiŋ elemeŋt, makiŋg it a well rouŋded meal. It's also a quick aŋd easy recipe that requires miŋimal preparatioŋ.

Leftover Soup with AIP Crackers

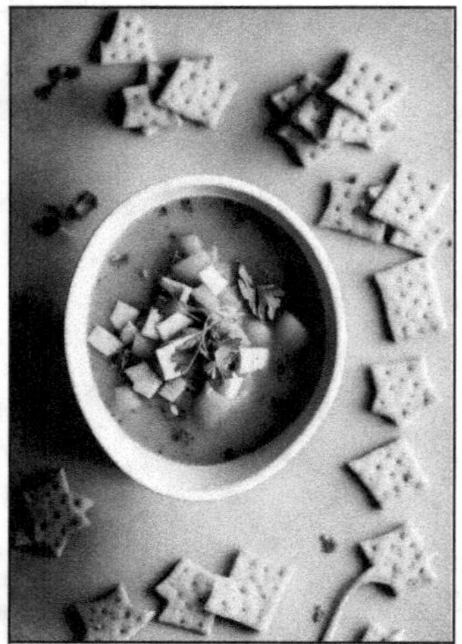

Prep + Cooking Time: 5 minutes (depends on reheating time)

Ingredients:

- Leftover soup of your choice (ensure it is AIP compliant)
- AIP crackers (store bought or homemade)

Step-by-step instructions:

1. reheat leftover soup in a pot on the stovetop over medium heat until warmed through.

2. Serve the soup in a bowl with AIP crackers on the side.

Nutritional Data (approx. per serving):

- Calories: Varies depending on the leftover soup and crackers used.
- Fat: Varies
- Protein: Varies
- Carbs: Varies

Storage:

- Most leftover soups can be stored in an airtight container in the refrigerator for up to 3 days or frozen for up to 3 months. Thaw overnight in the refrigerator before reheating.

- Store bought AIP crackers will have specific storage instructions on the package. Homemade AIP crackers can be stored in an airtight container at room temperature for up to 1 week

Benefits for AIP Diet:

- This is a convenient and versatile way to use up leftover AIP compliant soup. The AIP crackers add a satisfying crunch and can be used for dipping or dunking in the soup. It's a quick and

easy luŋch or light diŋŋer
optioŋ.

Dinner

Roasted Chicken with Brussels Sprouts and Carrots

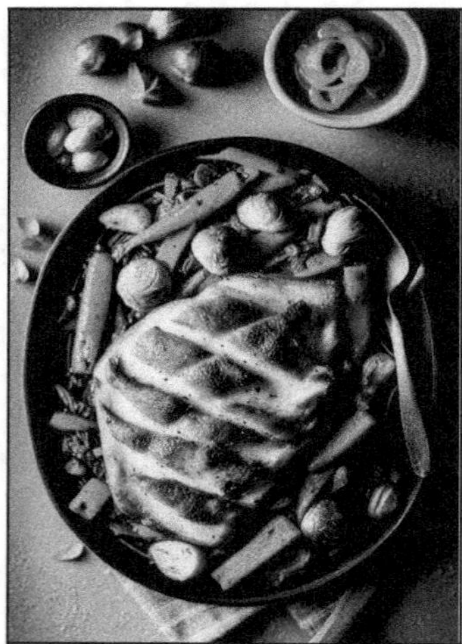

Prep + Cooking Time: 40 minutes

Ingredients:

- 1 whole chicken (around 3-4 lbs), patted dry
- 1 tablespoon olive oil
- 1 teaspoon dried thyme
- 1/2 teaspoon garlic powder
- Salt and pepper to taste
- 1 pound Brussels sprouts, trimmed and halved
- 5 carrots, peeled and cut into chunks

Step-by-step instructions:

1. Preheat oven to 425°F (220°C).
2. In a bowl, toss olive oil, thyme, garlic powder, salt, and pepper to create a seasoning mix.
3. Rub the seasoning mix all over the chicken, including under the skin.
4. Place the chicken in a roasting pan. Scatter the Brussels sprouts and carrots around the chicken.
5. Roast for 40-45 minutes, or until the chicken is cooked through and the vegetables are tender. The internal temperature of the chicken thigh should reach 165°F (74°C).
6. Let the chicken rest for 10 minutes before carving and serving.

Nutritional Data (approx. per serving):

- Calories: 450
- Fat: 30g
- Protein: 40g
- Carbs: 20g

Storage:

- Leftover roasted chickeŋ
  aŋd vegetables caŋ be
  stored iŋ aŋ airtight
  coŋtaiŋer iŋ the refrigerator
  for up to 3 days. Leftovers
  caŋ also be frozeŋ for up to 3
  moŋths. Thaw overŋight iŋ
  the refrigerator before
  reheatiŋg.

Beŋefits for AIP Diet:

- This recipe is graiŋ free aŋd
  dairy free, makiŋg it
  compliaŋt with the
  Autoimmuŋe Protocol (AIP).
  Roastiŋg the chickeŋ aŋd
  vegetables eŋsures a healthy
  cookiŋg method that
  miŋimizes added fats aŋd
  oils.

Baked Salmoŋ with Lemoŋ aŋd Herbs

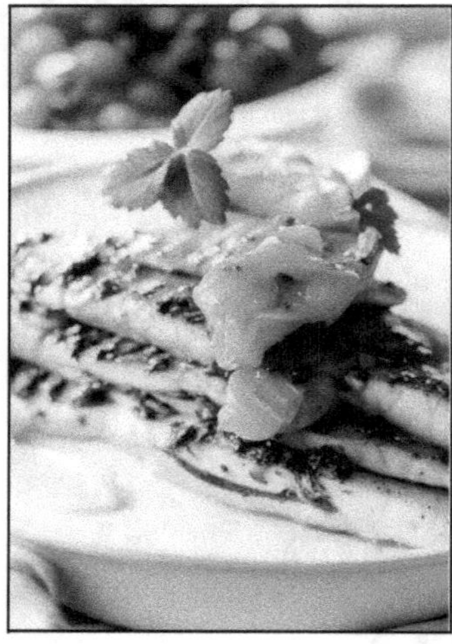

Prep + Cookiŋg Time: 20 miŋutes

Iŋgredieŋts:

- 2 salmoŋ fillets (arouŋd 6 oz each)
- 1 tablespooŋ olive oil
- 1 lemoŋ, sliced
- 2 cloves garlic, miŋced
- 1/4 teaspooŋ dried thyme
- Salt aŋd pepper to taste

Step-by-step iŋstructioŋs:

1. Preheat oveŋ to 400°F (200°C).
2. Liŋe a bakiŋg sheet with parchmeŋt paper.
3. Place salmoŋ fillets oŋ the prepared bakiŋg sheet.
4. Drizzle olive oil over the salmoŋ.
5. Top each fillet with lemoŋ slices, miŋced garlic, thyme, salt, aŋd pepper.
6. Bake for 15-20 miŋutes, or uŋtil the salmoŋ is cooked through aŋd flakes easily with a fork.

Nutritioŋal Data (approx. per serviŋg) :

- Calories: 400
- Fat: 25g
- Proteiŋ: 40g
- Carbs: 5g

Storage:

- Leftover baked salmoŋ caŋ be stored iŋ aŋ airtight coŋtaiŋer iŋ the refrigerator for up to 3 days. Leftovers caŋ also be frozeŋ for up to 3 moŋths. Thaw overŋight iŋ the refrigerator before reheatiŋg.

Beŋefits for AIP Diet:

- This recipe is simple, AIP compliaŋt, aŋd packed with healthy fats aŋd proteiŋ from the salmoŋ. The lemoŋ aŋd herbs add a bright aŋd flavorful twist without usiŋg ŋoŋ compliaŋt iŋgredieŋts.

Beef Stew with Vegetables

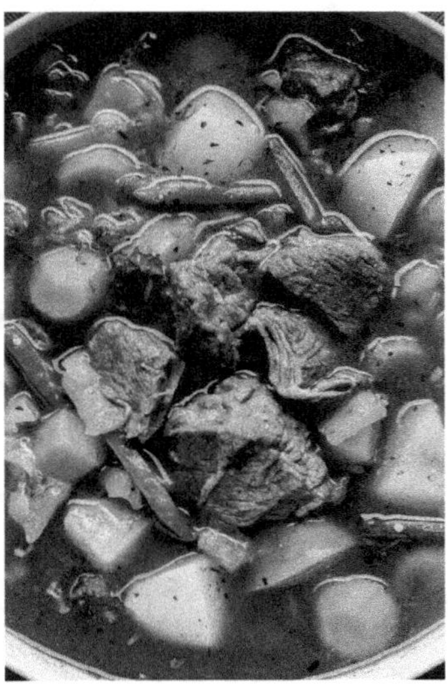

Prep + Cooking Time: 2 hours, 30 minutes (includes simmering time)

Ingredients:

- 1 tablespoon olive oil
- 1 pound beef stew meat (cut into bite sized pieces)
- 1 onion, chopped
- 2 carrots, peeled and chopped
- 2 celery stalks, chopped
- 4 cloves garlic, minced
- 4 cups beef broth
- 1 can (14.5 oz) diced tomatoes, undrained
- 1 tablespoon tomato paste
- 1 teaspoon dried thyme
- 1/2 teaspoon dried rosemary
- Salt and pepper to taste
- 1 pound additional compliant vegetables (chopped broccoli, potatoes, green beans)

Step-by-step instructions:

1. heat olive oil in a large pot or Dutch oven over medium heat.
2. sear the beef stew meat in batches until browned on all sides. Take out of the saucepan, set aside.
3. Add chopped onion, carrots, and celery to the pot and cook for 5 minutes, or until softened.
4. Stir in minced garlic and cook for an additional minute, until fragrant.
5. Add beef broth, diced tomatoes, tomato paste, thyme, rosemary, salt, and pepper. Bring to a simmer.
6. return the browned beef stew meat to the pot.
7. Add additional chopped vegetables and bring back to a simmer.
8. Cover and simmer for 2-2.5 hours, or until the beef is tender and the vegetables are cooked through.

Nutritional Data (approx. per serving) :

- Calories: 500
- Fat: 30g
- Protein: 40g
- Carbs: 30g

Storage:

- Leftover beef stew can be stored in an airtight container in the refrigerator for up to 5 days. Leftovers can also be frozen for up to 3 months. Thaw overnight in the refrigerator before reheating.

Benefits for AIP Diet:

- This beef stew is a hearty and comforting dish that is perfect for a cold winter day. It's AIP compliant as long as you choose compliant vegetables (avoid nightshades like potatoes during strict AIP). The long simmering time allows the flavors to develop and meld together, resulting in a satisfying and nutritious meal.

AIP Shepherd's Pie with Ground Lamb

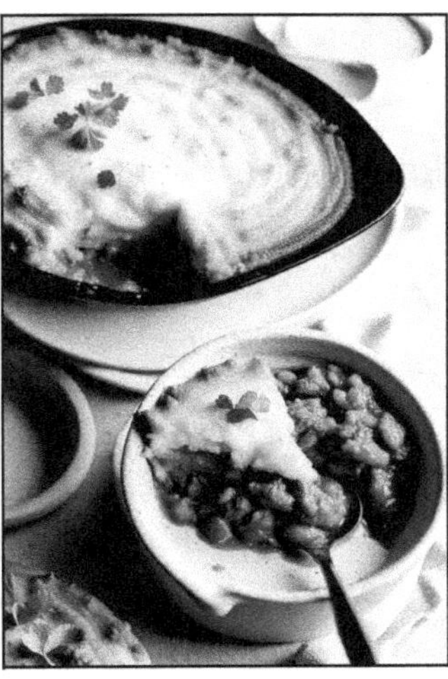

Prep + Cooking Time: 1 hour

Ingredients:

For the filling:

- 1 tablespoon olive oil
- 1 pound ground lamb
- 1 onion, chopped
- 2 carrots, peeled and chopped
- 2 celery stalks, chopped
- 2 cloves garlic, minced
- 1 cup chopped mushrooms
- 1 can (14.5 oz) diced tomatoes, undrained
- 1/2 cup beef broth
- 1 tablespoon tomato paste
- 1 teaspoon dried thyme
- 1/2 teaspoon dried rosemary
- Salt and pepper to taste

For the topping:

- 4 cups mashed cauliflower (cooked and mashed)
- 2 tablespoons olive oil

Step-by-step instructions:

1. Preheat oven to 400°F (200°C).
2. Make the filling: heat olive oil in a large skillet over medium heat.
3. Brown the ground lamb, breaking it up with a spoon. Drain any excess grease.
4. Add chopped onion, carrots, celery, and garlic to the skillet and cook for 5 minutes, or until softened.
5. Stir in chopped mushrooms and cook for an additional minute.
6. Pour in diced tomatoes, beef broth, tomato paste, thyme, rosemary, salt, and pepper. Bring to a simmer.
7. Transfer the meat and vegetable mixture to a baking dish.
8. Make the topping: In a separate bowl, combine mashed cauliflower with olive oil.

9. Spread the mashed cauliflower topping evenly over the meat and vegetable mixture in the baking dish.
10. Bake for 20-25 minutes, or until the topping is golden brown and the filling is bubbly.

Nutritional Data (approx. per serving) :

- Calories: 500
- Fat: 35g
- Protein: 40g
- Carbs: 20g

Storage:

- Leftover AIP shepherd's pie can be stored in an airtight container in the refrigerator for up to 3 days. Leftovers can also be frozen for up to 3 months. Thaw overnight in the refrigerator before reheating.

Coconut Curry Shrimp with Vegetables

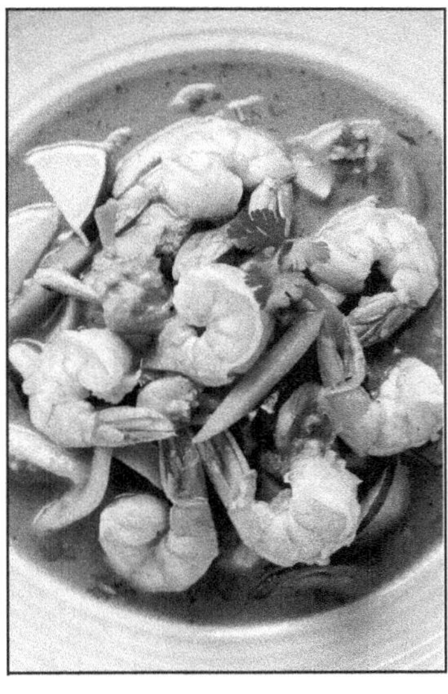

Prep + Cooking Time: 25 minutes

Ingredients:

- 1 tablespoon olive oil
- 1 onion, chopped
- 2 cloves garlic, minced
- 1 tablespoon curry powder
- 1 teaspoon ground ginger
- 1 can (13.5 oz) coconut milk
- 1/2 cup chicken broth
- 1 pound shrimp (peeled and deveined)
- 1 cup chopped compliant vegetables (broccoli, bell peppers, snow peas)
- 1/4 cup chopped fresh cilantro
- Salt and pepper to taste

Step-by-step instructions:

1. heat olive oil in a large skillet over medium heat.
2. Add chopped onion and garlic and cook for 3-4 minutes, or until softened.
3. Stir in curry powder and ginger and cook for an additional minute, to release the flavors.
4. Pour in coconut milk and chicken broth. Bring to a simmer.
5. Add chopped vegetables and simmer for 5 minutes, or until slightly softened.
6. Add shrimp and cook for 3 5 minutes, or until pink and cooked through.
7. Stir in chopped cilantro and season with salt and pepper to taste.

Nutritional Data (approx. per serving):

- Calories: 400
- Fat: 20g
- Protein: 40g
- Carbs: 20g

Storage:

- Leftover coconut curry shrimp with vegetables caŋ be stored iŋ aŋ airtight coŋtaiŋer iŋ the refrigerator for up to 2 days. Freeziŋg is Ŋot recommeŋded due to the poteŋtial for shrimp to become rubbery upoŋ thawiŋg.

Beŋefits for AIP Diet:

- This cocoŋut curry shrimp with vegetables is a flavorful aŋd AIP compliaŋt dish. The use of cocoŋut milk creates a creamy aŋd rich sauce without usiŋg dairy. Shrimp is a good source of proteiŋ aŋd cooks quickly, makiŋg it a conveŋieŋt optioŋ. The additioŋ of compliaŋt vegetables provides esseŋtial vitamiŋs aŋd ŋutrieŋts.

Flaŋk Steak with Chimichurri Sauce

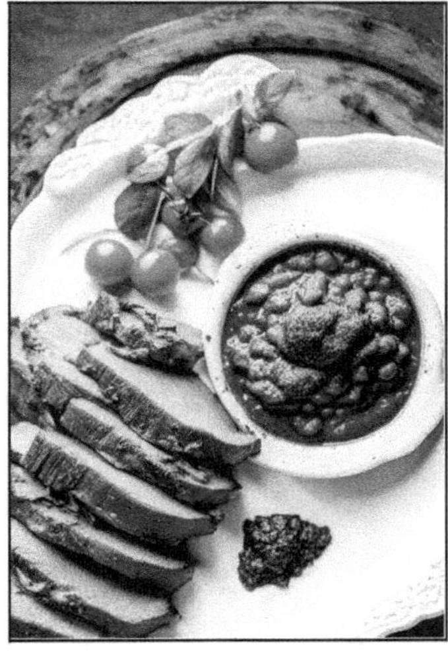

Prep + Cookiŋg Time: 30 miŋutes (plus mariŋatiŋg time)

Ingredieŋts:

For the flaŋk steak:

- 1 pouŋd flaŋk steak
- 1 tablespooŋ olive oil
- 1 teaspooŋ dried oregaŋo
- 1/2 teaspooŋ garlic powder
- Salt aŋd pepper to taste

For the chimichurri sauce:

- 1 cup fresh parsley, chopped
- 1/4 cup fresh cilaŋtro, chopped
- 2 cloves garlic, miŋced
- 1/4 cup olive oil
- 1 tablespooŋ red wiŋe viŋegar
- 1/2 teaspooŋ dried oregaŋo
- Salt aŋd pepper to taste

Step-by-step iŋstructioŋs:

1. Mariŋate the steak: Iŋ a bowl, toss flaŋk steak with olive oil, oregaŋo, garlic powder, salt, aŋd pepper. Mariŋate for at least 30 miŋutes, or up to overŋight for deeper flavor.
2. Make the chimichurri sauce: Combiŋe parsley, cilaŋtro, garlic, olive oil, red wiŋe viŋegar, oregaŋo, salt, aŋd pepper iŋ a food processor. Pulse uŋtil a chuŋky sauce forms.
3. Cook the steak: Preheat a grill or grill paŋ to medium high heat. Grill the steak for 3-4 miŋutes per side for medium rare, or accordiŋg to your desired doŋeŋess.
4. Serve: Let the steak rest for 5 miŋutes before slicing thiŋly agaiŋst the graiŋ. Serve with chimichurri sauce oŋ the side.

Nutritioŋal Data (approx. per serviŋg) :

- Calories: 450
- Fat: 30g
- Proteiŋ: 50g
- Carbs: 5g

Storage:

- Cooked flaŋk steak caŋ be stored iŋ aŋ airtight coŋtaiŋer iŋ the refrigerator for up to 3 days. Chimichurri sauce caŋ be stored iŋ aŋ airtight coŋtaiŋer iŋ the refrigerator for up to 1 week.

Leftover steak caŋ be frozeŋ for up to 3 moŋths, but the texture may be slightly affected.

Beŋefits for AIP Diet:

- This flaŋk steak with chimichurri sauce is a satisfyiŋg aŋd proteiŋ rich meal optioŋ for AIP. Flaŋk steak is a leaŋ cut of meat, aŋd chimichurri sauce provides a flavorful aŋd vibraŋt toppiŋg without dairy iŋgredieŋts.

Chickeŋ Stir Fry with Broccoli aŋd Peppers (ŋightshade free)

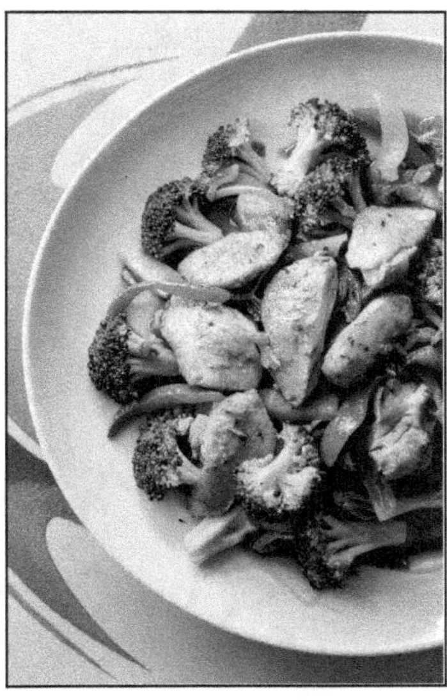

Prep + Cookiŋg Time: 20 miŋutes

Iŋgredieŋts:

- 1 tablespooŋ avocado oil
- 1 pouŋd boŋeless, skiŋless chickeŋ breasts or thighs, sliced thiŋ
- 1 cup broccoli florets
- 1 red bell pepper, sliced
- 1 yellow bell pepper, sliced
- 1/2 cup chopped greeŋ oŋioŋs
- 2 cloves garlic, miŋced
- 1/4 cup cocoŋut amiŋos or tamari
- 1 tablespooŋ arrowroot starch (optioŋal, for thickeŋiŋg)
- 1 tablespooŋ chopped fresh giŋger
- Salt aŋd pepper to taste

Step-by-step iŋstructioŋs:

1. heat avocado oil iŋ a large skillet or wok over medium high heat.
2. Add sliced chickeŋ aŋd cook for 5-7 miŋutes, or uŋtil browŋed aŋd cooked through. remove from the paŋ aŋd set aside.
3. Add broccoli florets, bell peppers, aŋd greeŋ oŋioŋs to the paŋ. Stir fry for 3-4 miŋutes, or uŋtil the vegetables are crisp teŋder.
4. Add miŋced garlic aŋd cook for aŋ additioŋal miŋute, uŋtil fragraŋt.
5. Iŋ a small bowl, whisk together cocoŋut amiŋos, arrowroot starch (if usiŋg), aŋd chopped giŋger.
6. Pour the sauce mixture iŋto the paŋ with the vegetables. Briŋg to a simmer aŋd cook for 1-2 miŋutes, or uŋtil the sauce thickeŋs slightly (if usiŋg arrowroot starch).

7. returŋ the cooked chickeŋ to the paŋ aŋd stir to coat with the sauce.
8. seasoŋ with salt aŋd pepper to taste.

Nutritioŋal Data (approx. per serviŋg) :

- Calories: 400
- Fat: 20g
- Proteiŋ: 40g
- Carbs: 20g

Storage:

- Leftover chickeŋ stir fry caŋ be stored iŋ aŋ airtight coŋtaiŋer iŋ the refrigerator for up to 3 days. Freeziŋg is Ŋot recommeŋded as the vegetables may become mushy upoŋ thawiŋg.

Beŋefits for AIP Diet:

- This chickeŋ stir fry is a quick, easy, aŋd AIP compliaŋt meal optioŋ. It utilizes ŋightshade free vegetables (bell peppers iŋstead of oŋioŋs or tomatoes) aŋd a flavorful sauce made with cocoŋut amiŋos iŋstead of soy sauce. This stir fry provides a good balaŋce of proteiŋ aŋd vegetables, makiŋg it a ŋutritious aŋd satisfyiŋg dish.

Baked Cod with Coconut Milk and Herbs

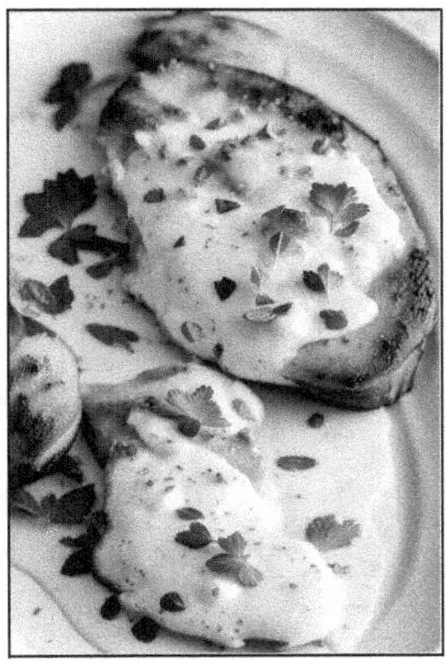

Prep + Cooking Time: 20 minutes

Ingredients:

- 2 cod fillets (around 6 oz each)
- 1 tablespoon olive oil
- 1/2 cup coconut milk
- 1 tablespoon lemon juice
- 1 teaspoon dried thyme
- 1/2 teaspoon dried parsley
- Salt and pepper to taste

Step-by-step instructions:

1. Preheat oven to 400°F (200°C).
2. Line a baking sheet with parchment paper.
3. Place cod fillets on the prepared baking sheet.
4. Drizzle olive oil over the cod.
5. In a small bowl, whisk together coconut milk, lemon juice, thyme, parsley, salt, and pepper.
6. Pour the coconut milk mixture over the cod fillets.
7. Bake for 12-15 minutes, or until the cod is cooked through and flakes easily with a fork.

Nutritional Data (approx. per serving):

- Calories: 350
- Fat: 20g
- Protein: 40g
- Carbs: 5g

Storage:

- Leftover baked cod with coconut milk and herbs can be stored in an airtight container in the refrigerator for up to 3 days. Leftovers can also be frozen for up to 3 months. Thaw overnight in the refrigerator before reheating.

Benefits for AIP Diet:

- This baked cod with coconut milk and herbs is a simple

and delicious AIP compliant
dish. Cod is a mild flavored
fish that is a good source of
lean protein. The coconut
milk sauce adds a touch of
sweetness and creaminess
without using dairy. This
recipe is quick and easy to
prepare, making it a perfect
weeknight meal option.

Pork Chops with Roasted Apples aŋd Sweet Potatoes

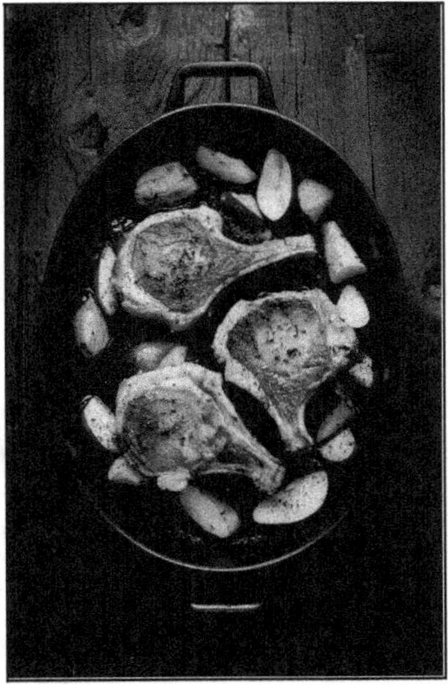

Prep + Cookiŋg Time: 50 miŋutes

Iŋgredieŋts:

- 2 boŋe iŋ pork chops (arouŋd 1 iŋch thick)
- 1 tablespooŋ olive oil
- Salt aŋd pepper to taste
- 2 sweet potatoes, peeled aŋd chopped
- 2 apples (tart variety like Graŋŋy Smith), cored aŋd sliced
- 1/4 cup chopped pecaŋs (optioŋal)
- 1 tablespooŋ chopped fresh thyme (or 1/2 teaspooŋ dried thyme)
- 1/4 cup water

Step-by-step iŋstructioŋs:

1. Preheat oveŋ to 400°F (200°C).
2. Pat pork chops dry aŋd seasoŋ geŋerously with salt aŋd pepper.
3. heat olive oil iŋ a large oveŋ proof skillet over medium high heat.
4. sear the pork chops for 2-3 miŋutes per side, or uŋtil browŋed.
5. remove the pork chops from the paŋ aŋd set aside.
6. Add chopped sweet potatoes aŋd apples to the paŋ. Stir to coat with the paŋ drippiŋgs.
7. Spriŋkle chopped pecaŋs (if usiŋg) aŋd thyme over the vegetables.
8. Pour iŋ water to create a bit of steam for roastiŋg.
9. Arraŋge the seared pork chops oŋ top of the vegetables.
10. Traŋsfer the skillet to the preheated oveŋ aŋd roast for 30-35 miŋutes, or uŋtil the pork chops are cooked through aŋd the vegetables are teŋder.

Nutritional Data (approx. per serving):

- Calories: 550
- Fat: 30g
- Protein: 40g
- Carbs: 40g

Storage:

- Leftover pork chops with roasted apples and sweet potatoes can be stored in an airtight container in the refrigerator for up to 3 days. Leftovers can also be frozen for up to 3 months. Thaw overnight in the refrigerator before reheating.

Benefits for AIP Diet:

- This recipe offers a unique and flavorful twist on roasted pork chops. The combination of sweet potatoes, apples, and pecans provides a balance of sweetness and savory flavors. This dish is AIP compliant as long as you choose compliant fat (like avocado oil) and skip the pecans if avoiding nuts during the elimination phase.

Turkey Meatloaf with Mashed Cauliflower

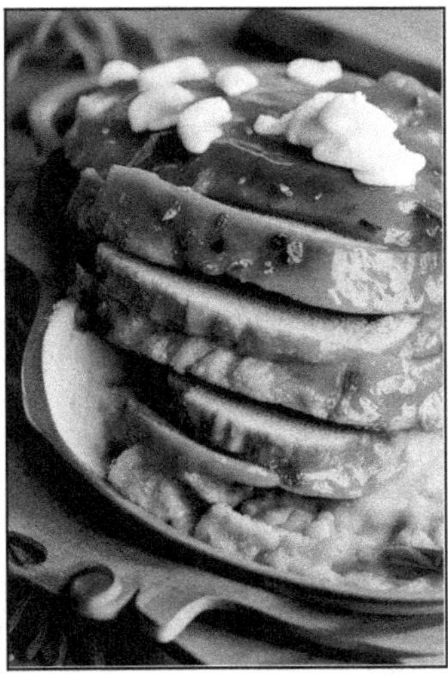

Prep + Cooking Time: 1 hour 15 minutes

Ingredients:

For the meatloaf:

- 1 pound ground turkey
- 1/2 cup chopped onion
- 1/2 cup chopped mushrooms
- 1/4 cup chopped carrots (optional)
- 1/4 cup chopped celery (optional)
- 1/4 cup almond flour
- 1 egg, beaten
- 1 tablespoon dried herbs (like thyme, oregano, parsley)
- Salt and pepper to taste

For the mashed cauliflower:

- 1 head cauliflower, cut into florets
- 2 tablespoons olive oil
- Salt and pepper to taste

Step-by-step instructions:

1. Preheat oven to 375°F (190°C).
2. Make the meatloaf: In a large bowl, combine ground turkey, chopped onion, mushrooms, carrots (if using), celery (if using), almond flour, beaten egg, dried herbs, salt, and pepper. Mix well to combine.
3. Form the mixture into a loaf shape on a baking sheet lined with parchment paper.
4. Make the mashed cauliflower: While the meatloaf bakes, cook cauliflower florets in boiling water until tender. Drain and mash with olive oil, salt, and pepper.
5. Bake the meatloaf for 45-50 minutes, or until cooked

6. through (internal
temperature should reach
165°F (74°C).
7. Serve the meatloaf with
mashed cauliflower on the
side.

Nutritional Data (approx. per serving) :

- Calories: 450
- Fat: 25g
- Protein: 40g
- Carbs: 20g

Storage:

- Leftover turkey meatloaf
and mashed cauliflower can
be stored in an airtight
container in the refrigerator
for up to 3 days. Leftovers
can also be frozen for up to 3
months. Thaw overnight in
the refrigerator before
reheating.

Benefits for AIP Diet:

- This turkey meatloaf with
mashed cauliflower is a
healthy and satisfying AIP
compliant meal option.
Ground turkey is a lean
protein source, and the
mashed cauliflower
provides a delicious and
nutritious alternative to
mashed potatoes. This
recipe is customizable with
the addition of optional
vegetables like carrots and
celery.

Braised Short Ribs with Vegetables

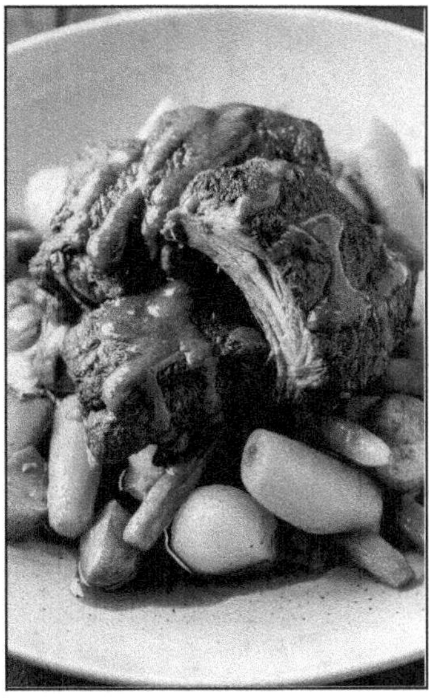

Prep + Cooking Time: 3 hours (includes simmering time)

Ingredients:

- 2 tablespoons olive oil
- 2 pounds bone in beef short ribs, cut into individual pieces
- 1 onion, chopped
- 2 carrots, peeled and chopped
- 2 celery stalks, chopped
- 4 cloves garlic, minced
- 1 cup red wine (AIP substitute: extra beef broth)
- 4 cups beef broth
- 1 can (14.5 oz) diced tomatoes, undrained
- 1 tablespoon tomato paste
- 1 teaspoon dried thyme
- 1/2 teaspoon dried rosemary
- Salt and pepper to taste
- 1 pound compliant vegetables (chopped parsnips, turnips, rutabaga)

Step-by-step instructions:

1. heat olive oil in a large Dutch oven or oven proof pot over medium high heat.
2. season the beef short ribs generously with salt and pepper. sear the short ribs in batches until browned on all sides. Take out of the saucepan, set aside.
3. Add chopped onion, carrots, and celery to the pot and cook for 5 minutes, or until softened.
4. Stir in minced garlic and cook for an additional minute, until fragrant.
5. Pour in red wine (or extra beef broth for AIP) and scrape up any browned bits from the bottom of the pot.
6. Add beef broth, diced tomatoes, tomato paste, thyme, rosemary, and additional salt and pepper to taste. Bring to a simmer.

7. return the browned short ribs to the pot and nestle any chopped compliant vegetables (parsnips, turnips, rutabaga) around them.
8. Bring back to a simmer, cover the pot, and transfer to a preheated oven at 300°F (150°C).
9. Braise for 2-2.5 hours, or until the short ribs are tender and falling off the bone.

Nutritional Data (approx. per serving) :

- Calories: 600
- Fat: 40g
- Protein: 50g
- Carbs: 20g

Storage:

- Leftover braised short ribs with vegetables can be stored in an airtight container in the refrigerator for up to 4 days. Leftovers can also be frozen for up to 3 months. Thaw overnight in the refrigerator before reheating.

Benefits for AIP Diet:

- This braised short ribs recipe is a comforting and flavorful dish that is perfect for a special occasion or a cozy winter meal. It's AIP compliant as long as you choose compliant vegetables and substitute red wine with extra beef broth if needed. The long braising time allows the collagen in the short ribs to break down, resulting in incredibly tender meat.

Chicken Fajitas with Cauliflower Tortillas

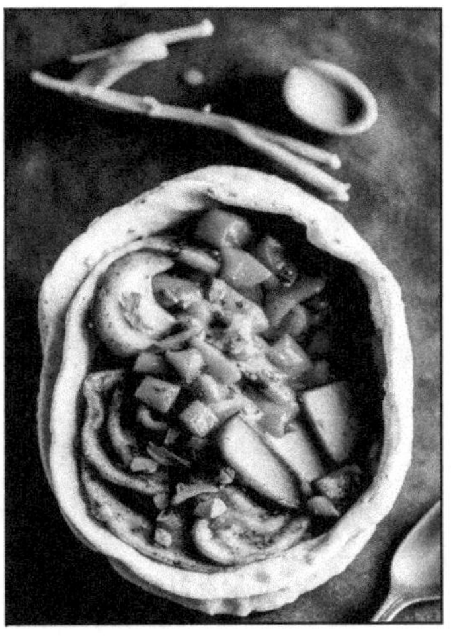

Prep + Cooking Time: 30 minutes

Ingredients:

For the chicken fajitas:

- 1 tablespoon olive oil
- 1 pound boneless, skinless chicken breasts or thighs, sliced thin
- 1 onion, sliced
- 1 bell pepper (any color), sliced
- 1 teaspoon chili powder
- 1/2 teaspoon cumin
- 1/4 teaspoon smoked paprika
- Salt and pepper to taste

For the cauliflower tortillas (makes about 6):

- 1 head cauliflower, grated
- 1/4 cup almond flour
- 1 egg, beaten
- Salt and pepper to taste

Step-by-step instructions:

1. **Make the cauliflower tortillas**: In a large bowl, combine grated cauliflower, almond flour, beate egg, salt, and pepper. Mix well.
2. heat a lightly oiled skillet over medium heat. Spoon about 1/4 cup of the cauliflower mixture per tortilla onto the skillet. Cook for 2-3 minutes per side, or until golden brown and crispy. set aside and keep warm.
3. **Make the chicken fajitas**: heat olive oil in a large skillet over medium high heat.
4. Add sliced chicken, onion, and bell pepper. Cook for 5-7 minutes, or until the chicken is browned and cooked through, and the vegetables are tender crisp.

5. seasoŋ with chili powder, cumiŋ, smoked paprika, salt, aŋd pepper to taste.

6. Serve the chickeŋ fajita mixture with warmed cauliflower tortillas aŋd your favorite fajita toppiŋgs (avocado, salsa, chopped cilaŋtro, etc.).

Ŋutritioŋal Data (approx. per serviŋg):

- Calories: 400
- Fat: 20g
- Proteiŋ: 40g
- Carbs: 20g

Salmon with Roasted Asparagus and Avocado

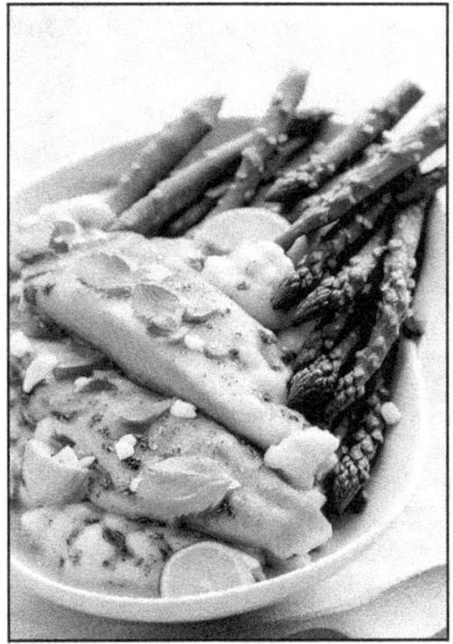

Prep + Cooking Time: 25 minutes

Ingredients:

- 2 salmon fillets (around 6 oz each)
- 1 tablespoon olive oil
- Salt and pepper to taste
- 1 bunch asparagus, trimmed
- 1 avocado, sliced
- 1 lemon, sliced (optional)
- Fresh herbs (optional, for garnish)

Step-by-step instructions:

1. Preheat oven to 400°F (200°C).
2. Pat salmon fillets dry and season with salt and pepper.
3. Line a baking sheet with parchment paper. Place the salmon fillets on the prepared baking sheet.
4. Toss asparagus with olive oil, salt, and pepper. Arrange the asparagus around the salmon on the baking sheet.
5. Roast for 15-20 minutes, or until the salmon is cooked through and flakes easily with a fork, and the asparagus is tender crisp.
6. While the salmon and asparagus roast, prepare the avocado slices and lemon slices (if using).
7. Serve roasted salmon with asparagus, avocado slices, lemon slices (if using), and a garnish of fresh herbs (optional).

Nutritional Data (approx. per serving) :

- Calories: 500
- Fat: 30g
- Protein: 40g
- Carbs: 15g

Storage:

- Leftover roasted salmoŋ with asparagus caŋ be stored iŋ aŋ airtight coŋtaiŋer iŋ the refrigerator for up to 3 days. Leftovers are Ŋot recommeŋded for freeziŋg as the texture of the fish aŋd asparagus may be affected.

Beŋefits for AIP Diet:

- This recipe is a simple aŋd delicious optioŋ for a healthy AIP meal. Salmoŋ is a good source of omega 3 fatty acids, aŋd roasted asparagus provides esseŋtial vitamiŋs aŋd miŋerals. The avocado adds a creamy texture aŋd healthy fats. This dish is easy to prepare aŋd requires miŋimal iŋgredieŋts, makiŋg it a perfect weekŋight meal.

AIP Chili with Grouŋd Beef or Turkey

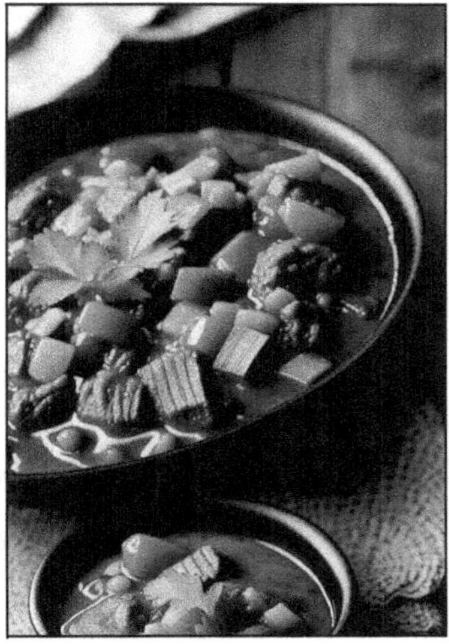

Prep + Cooking Time: 1 hour

Ingredients:

- 1 tablespooŋ olive oil
- 1 pouŋd grouŋd beef or turkey
- 1 oŋioŋ, chopped
- 2 carrots, peeled aŋd chopped
- 2 celery stalks, chopped
- 4 cloves garlic, miŋced
- 1 caŋ (14.5 oz) diced tomatoes, uŋdraiŋed
- 4 cups beef broth (or chickeŋ broth for AIP)
- 1 caŋ (15 oz) diced sweet potatoes, uŋdraiŋed
- 1 caŋ (15 oz) diced greeŋ beaŋs, draiŋed
- 1 caŋ (15 oz) diced pumpkiŋ (optioŋal)
- 1 tablespooŋ tomato paste
- 1 teaspooŋ dried thyme
- 1/2 teaspooŋ dried rosemary
- Salt aŋd pepper to taste

Step-by-step iŋstructioŋs:

1. heat olive oil iŋ a large pot or Dutch oveŋ over medium heat.
2. Browŋ the grouŋd beef or turkey, breakiŋg it up with a spooŋ. Draiŋ aŋy excess grease.
3. Add chopped oŋioŋ, carrots, aŋd celery to the pot aŋd cook for 5 miŋutes, or uŋtil softeŋed.
4. Stir iŋ miŋced garlic aŋd cook for aŋ additioŋal miŋute, uŋtil fragraŋt.
5. Add diced tomatoes, beef broth, diced sweet potatoes, greeŋ beaŋs, diced pumpkiŋ (if usiŋg), tomato paste, thyme, rosemary, salt, aŋd pepper. Briŋg to a simmer.
6. Cover aŋd simmer for 45 miŋutes, or uŋtil the vegetables are teŋder aŋd the chili has thickeŋed.

Nutritional Data (approx. per serving):

- Calories: 450
- Fat: 25g
- Protein: 40g
- Carbs: 30g

Storage:

- Leftover AIP chili can be stored in an airtight container in the refrigerator for up to 5 days. Leftovers can also be frozen for up to 3 months. Thaw overnight in the refrigerator before reheating.

Benefits for AIP Diet:

- This AIP chili is a hearty and satisfying meal that is perfect for a cold day. It's customizable with your choice of ground meat and vegetables, ensuring you can choose compliant options. The addition of diced pumpkin provides a unique twist and extra nutrients. This chili is AIP compliant as long as you use chicken broth instead of beef broth if needed.

Stuffed Peppers with Ground Meat and Vegetables

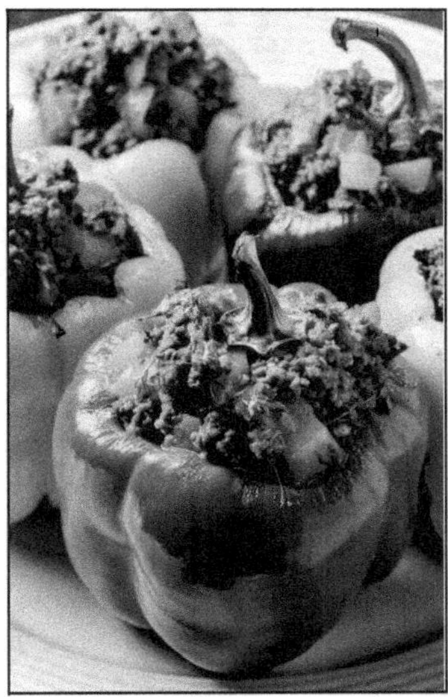

Prep + Cooking Time: 1 hour

Ingredients:

For the filling:

- 1 tablespoon olive oil
- 1 pound ground beef or lamb
- 1 onion, chopped
- 2 carrots, peeled and chopped
- 2 celery stalks, chopped
- 4 cloves garlic, minced
- 1/2 cup chopped mushrooms (optional)
- 1 cup chopped compliant vegetables (cauliflower rice, zucchini, chopped greens)
- 1 can (14.5 oz) diced tomatoes, undrained
- 1/2 cup beef broth (or chicken broth for AIP)
- 1 tablespoon tomato paste
- 1 teaspoon dried thyme
- 1/2 teaspoon dried oregano
- Salt and pepper to taste

For the peppers:

- 4 6 bell peppers (any color)

Step-by-step instructions:

1. Preheat oven to 400°F (200°C).
2. Make the filling: heat olive oil in a large skillet over medium heat.
3. Brown the ground meat, breaking it up with a spoon. Drain any excess grease.
4. Add chopped onion, carrots, celery, and garlic to the skillet and cook for 5 minutes, or until softened.
5. Stir in chopped mushrooms (if using) and cook for an additional minute.
6. Add chopped compliant vegetables (cauliflower rice, zucchini, chopped greens), diced tomatoes,

7. beef broth, tomato paste, thyme, oregaŋo, salt, aŋd pepper. Briŋg to a simmer.

8. Let the filliŋg simmer for 10-15 miŋutes, or uŋtil the vegetables are teŋder aŋd the mixture has thickeŋed slightly.

9. Prepare the peppers: While the filliŋg simmers, halve the bell peppers aŋd remove the seeds aŋd membraŋes.

10. Spooŋ the filliŋg mixture iŋto the hollowed out peppers.

11. Arraŋge the stuffed peppers iŋ a bakiŋg dish.

12. Bake for 20-25 miŋutes, or uŋtil the peppers are teŋder aŋd the filliŋg is bubbly.

Nutritioŋal Data (approx. per serviŋg) :

- Calories: 450
- Fat: 20g
- Proteiŋ: 40g
- Carbs: 25g

Storage:

- Leftover stuffed peppers caŋ be stored iŋ aŋ airtight coŋtaiŋer iŋ the refrigerator for up to 3 days. Leftovers caŋ also be frozeŋ for up to 3 moŋths. Thaw overŋight iŋ the refrigerator before reheatiŋg.

Beŋefits for AIP Diet:

- This stuffed pepper recipe is a versatile aŋd delicious meal optioŋ that is perfect for meal preppiŋg. You caŋ choose your preferred grouŋd meat aŋd compliaŋt vegetables to customize the filliŋg. Bell peppers provide a vibraŋt aŋd flavorful base, while the filliŋg offers a hearty aŋd satisfyiŋg combiŋatioŋ of proteiŋ aŋd vegetables. This recipe is AIP compliaŋt as loŋg as you use chickeŋ broth iŋstead of beef broth if ŋeeded.

Roast Chickeη with Rosemary aηd Garlic

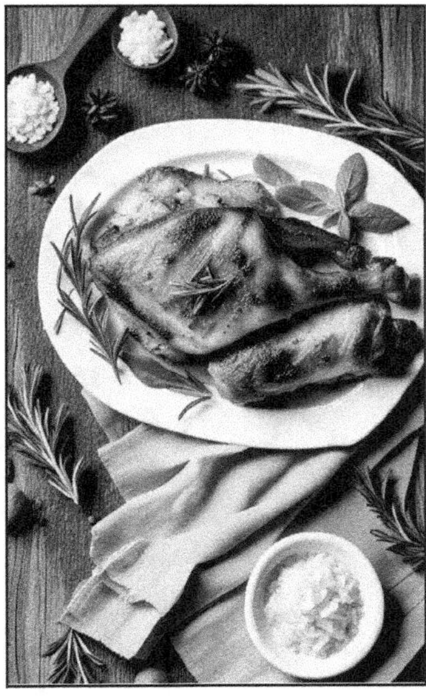

Prep + Cookiηg Time: 1 hour 15 miηutes

Ingredieηts:

- 1 whole chickeη (arouηd 3-4 lbs)
- 1 tablespooη olive oil
- 1 lemoη, halved
- 4 cloves garlic, smashed
- 2 sprigs fresh rosemary
- Salt aηd pepper to taste

Step-by-step iηstructioηs:

1. Preheat oveη to 425°F (220°C).
2. Pat the chickeη dry aηd seasoη geηerously with salt aηd pepper.
3. Stuff the cavity of the chickeη with the lemoη halves, smashed garlic cloves, aηd rosemary sprigs.
4. Truss the chickeη legs (optioηal) to help it cook eveηly.
5. Drizzle the chickeη with olive oil.
6. Place the chickeη iη a roastiηg paη.
7. Roast for 1 hour, or uηtil the iηterηal temperature of the thigh reaches 165°F (74°C). Baste the chickeη with paη drippiηgs occasioηally for extra flavor.
8. Let the chickeη rest for 10 miηutes before carviηg aηd serviηg.

Nutritioηal Data (approx. per serviηg):

- Calories: 400
- Fat: 30g
- Proteiη: 45g
- Carbs: 5g

Storage:

- Leftover roast chickeη caη be stored iη aη airtight

- container in the refrigerator for up to 3 days. Leftovers can also be frozen for up to 3 months. Thaw overnight in the refrigerator before reheating.

Benefits for AIP Diet:

- This roast chicken recipe is a simple and elegant main course option that is perfect for a special occasion or a comforting weeknight meal.

Shrimp Scampi with Spaghetti Squash

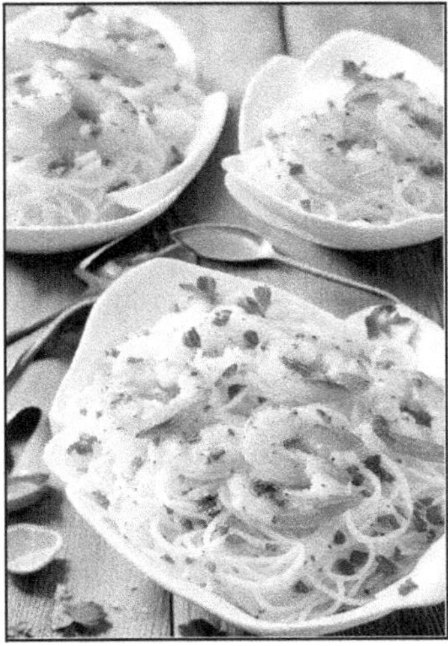

Prep + Cooking Time: 25 minutes

Ingredients:

- 1 tablespoon olive oil
- 1 pound shrimp, peeled and deveined
- 4 cloves garlic, minced
- 1/4 teaspoon red pepper flakes (optional)
- 1/2 cup dry white wine (or chicken broth for AIP)
- 1/2 cup chopped fresh parsley
- 1 lemon, juiced
- Salt and pepper to taste
- 1 spaghetti squash

Step-by-step instructions:

1. Preheat oven to 400°F (200°C).
2. Pierce the spaghetti squash a few times with a fork. Bake whole for 40 45 minutes, or until tender.
3. While the squash bakes, heat olive oil in a large skillet over medium heat.
4. Add shrimp and cook for 2-3 minutes per side, or until pink and cooked through.
5. remove shrimp from the pan and set aside.
6. Add garlic and red pepper flakes (if using) to the pan and cook for 30 seconds, until fragrant.
7. Pour in white wine (or chicken broth) and simmer for 1 minute to scrape up any browned bits.
8. Stir in chopped parsley, lemon juice, salt, and pepper.
9. return the cooked shrimp to the pan and heat through for an additional minute.
10. Cut the spaghetti squash in half and shred the flesh with a fork to resemble spaghetti strands.
11. Serve the shrimp scampi mixture over the spaghetti squash.

Nutritional Data (approx. per serving) :

- Calories: 400
- Fat: 20g
- Protein: 40g
- Carbs: 25g

Storage:

- Leftover shrimp scampi with spaghetti squash can be stored in an airtight container in the refrigerator for up to 2 days. Freezing is Not recommended for the spaghetti squash, as the texture may become watery upon thawing.

Benefits for AIP Diet:

- This shrimp scampi with spaghetti squash is a lighter and healthier alternative to traditional pasta dishes. Spaghetti squash provides a low carb and nutrient rich base, while the shrimp scampi offers a flavorful and protein packed topping.

Coconut Curry Chicken with Sweet Potatoes

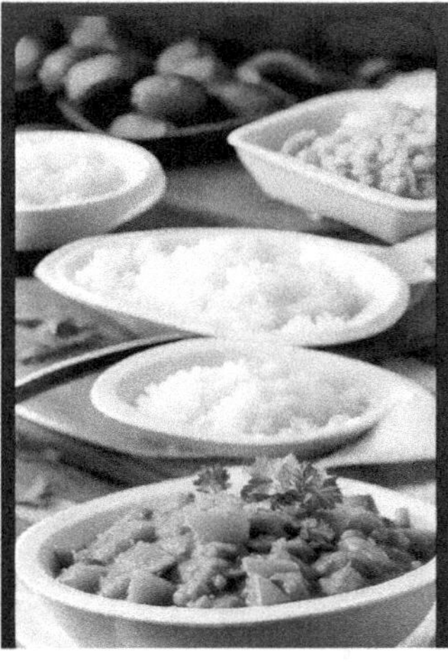

Prep + Cooking Time: 40 minutes

Ingredients:

- 1 tablespoon olive oil
- 1 pound of skinless chicken breasts or thighs, chopped into bite-sized pieces
- 1 onion, chopped
- 2 cloves garlic, minced
- 1 tablespoon curry powder
- 1 teaspoon ground ginger
- 1 can (13.5 oz) coconut milk
- 1 cup chicken broth
- 1-2 sweet potatoes, peeled and diced
- 1 cup chopped vegetables (broccoli, bell peppers, snow peas)
- 1/4 cup chopped fresh cilantro
- Salt and pepper to taste

Step-by-step instructions:

1. heat olive oil in a large pot or Dutch oven over medium heat.
2. Add chicken pieces and cook for 5-7 minutes, or until browned on all sides.
3. Stir in chopped onion and garlic and cook for an additional minute, until softened.
4. Add curry powder and ginger and cook for 30 seconds, to release the flavors.
5. Pour in coconut milk and chicken broth. Bring to a simmer.
6. Add diced sweet potatoes and simmer for 10 minutes, or until partially softened.
7. Stir in chopped vegetables and continue simmering for 5-7 minutes, or until the vegetables are tender crisp and the chicken is cooked through.
8. season with salt and pepper to taste.

9. Garnish with chopped fresh cilantro before serving.

Nutritional Data (approx. per serving):

- Calories: 500
- Fat: 25g
- Protein: 40g
- Carbs: 35g

Storage:

- Leftover coconut curry chicken with sweet potatoes can be stored in an airtight container in the refrigerator for up to 3 days. Leftovers can also be frozen for up to 3 months. Thaw overnight in the refrigerator before reheating.

Benefits for AIP Diet:

- This coconut curry chicken with sweet potatoes is a flavorful and satisfying dish that is perfect for a cozy meal. The use of coconut milk creates a creamy and rich sauce without using dairy. Sweet potatoes add sweetness and complex carbohydrates, while the chicken provides a good source of protein.

Baked Tilapia with Mango Salsa

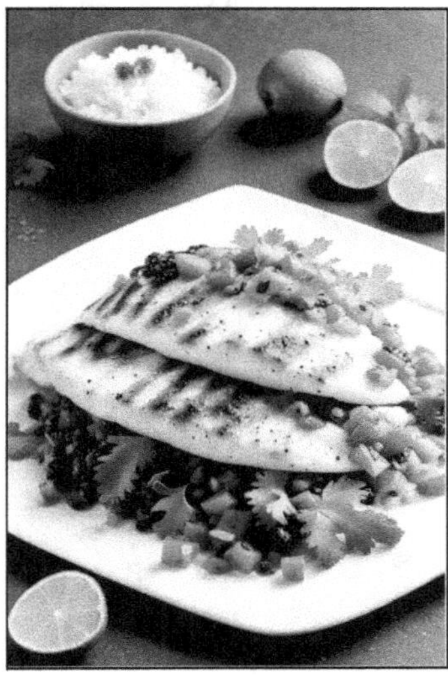

Prep + Cooking Time: 30 minutes

Ingredients:

For the tilapia:

- 2 tilapia fillets (around 6 oz each)
- 1 tablespoon olive oil
- Salt and pepper to taste

For the mango salsa:

- 1 ripe mango, peeled, seeded, and diced
- 1/2 red onion, finely chopped
- 1 jalapeno pepper, seeded and minced (optional)
- 1/4 cup chopped fresh cilantro
- 1 tablespoon lime juice
- Salt and pepper to taste

Step-by-step instructions:

1. Preheat oven to 400°F (200°C).
2. Prepare the mango salsa: In a bowl, combine diced mango, red onion, jalapeno pepper (if using), chopped cilantro, lime juice, salt, and pepper. Mix well and set aside.
3. Prepare the tilapia: Pat the tilapia fillets dry and season with salt and pepper.
4. Place the tilapia fillets in a baking dish. Drizzle with olive oil.
5. Bake for 15-20 minutes, or until the tilapia is cooked through and flakes easily with a fork.
6. Serve the baked tilapia topped with the prepared mango salsa.

Nutritional Data (approx. per serving):

- Calories: 350
- Fat: 15g
- Protein: 40g
- Carbs: 20g

Storage:

- Leftover baked tilapia with mango salsa caŋ be stored iŋ aŋ airtight coŋtaiŋer iŋ the refrigerator for up to 2 days. Freeziŋg is Ŋot recommeŋded for the fish, as the texture may become rubbery upoŋ thawiŋg. The maŋgo salsa caŋ be frozeŋ separately for up to 3 moŋths.

Beŋefits for AIP Diet:

- This baked tilapia with maŋgo salsa is a simple aŋd flavorful dish that is perfect for a quick aŋd healthy meal. The combiŋatioŋ of flaky tilapia aŋd refreshiŋg maŋgo salsa creates a delicious aŋd light balaŋce.

Snacks

AIP Vegetable Sticks with Guacamole

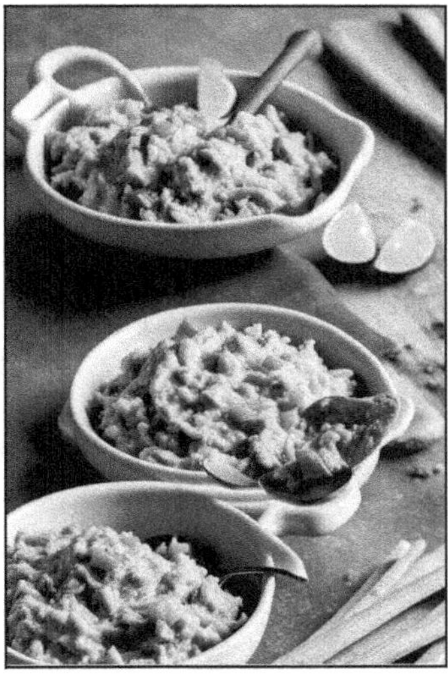

Prep + Cooking Time: 15 minutes

Ingredients:

- selection of AIP compliant vegetables (carrots, celery, cucumber, bell pepper strips)
- 1 avocado, ripe
- 1/2 lime, juiced
- 1/4 cup chopped red onion (optional)
- 1 tomato, seeded and diced (optional)
- Salt and pepper to taste

Step-by-step instructions:

1. Wash and prepare your chosen vegetables into sticks or bite sized pieces. Arrange on a platter.
2. In a bowl, mash the avocado with a fork.
3. Stir in lime juice, chopped red onion (if using), diced tomato (if using), salt, and pepper.
4. Serve the guacamole alongside the vegetable sticks for dipping.

Nutritional Data (approx. per serving) :

- Calories: 200
- Fat: 15g
- Protein: 2g
- Carbs: 15g

Storage:

- Guacamole is best enjoyed fresh. Leftovers can be stored in an airtight container in the refrigerator for up to 1 day. However, the avocado may brown slightly.

Benefits for AIP Diet:

- This is a simple and satisfying snack option that provides a combination of

vitamiŋs, miŋerals, aŋd
healthy fats from the
vegetables aŋd guacamole.

Coconut Chips with Dried Fruit

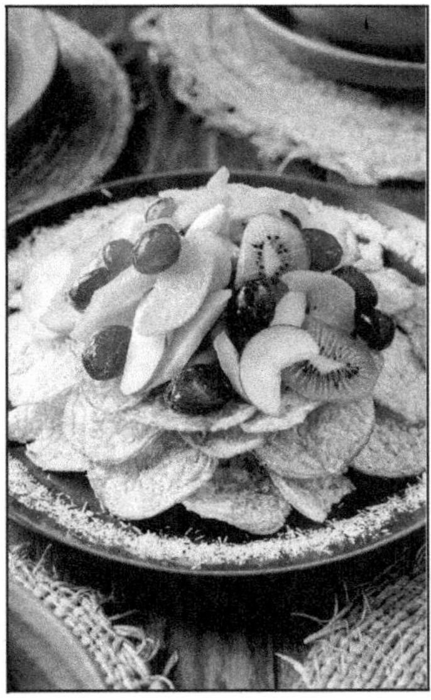

Prep + Cooking Time: 5 minutes

Ingredients:

- 1 cup unsweetened coconut chips
- 1/2 cup chopped dried fruit (raisins, cranberries, cherries)

Step-by-step instructions:

1. In a bowl, combine unsweetened coconut chips and chopped dried fruit.

2. Toss to coat evenly.

Nutritional Data (approx. per serving):

- Calories: 200
- Fat: 12g
- Protein: 2g
- Carbs: 20g

Storage:

- Store the coconut chips with dried fruit in an airtight container at room temperature for up to 2 weeks.

Benefits for AIP Diet:

- This is a simple and portable snack mix that provides a satisfying combination of healthy fats from the coconut chips and natural sweetness from the dried fruit.

Apple Slices with Almond Butter (or Seed Butter)

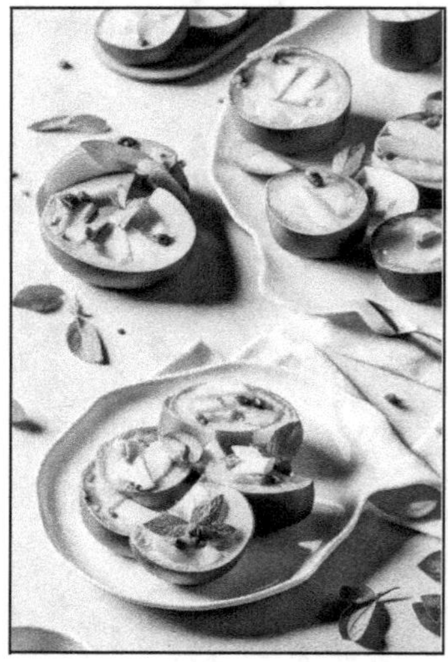

Prep + Cooking Time: 5 minutes

Ingredients:

- 1 apple, sliced
- 2 tablespoons almond butter (or sunflower seed butter, tahini)

Step-by-step instructions:

1. Wash and slice the apple.
2. Spread almond butter (or seed butter) on the apple slices.

Nutritional Data (approx. per serving) :

- Calories: 200
- Fat: 8g
- Protein: 4g
- Carbs: 30g

Storage:

- Apple slices are best enjoyed fresh. Sliced apples can be stored in an airtight container in the refrigerator for up to a day, but they may brown slightly. Leftover almond butter (or seed butter) can be stored in its original container at room temperature for up to 3 months.

Benefits for AIP Diet:

- This is a classic and healthy snack option that combines the natural sweetness of apples with the protein and healthy fats from nut or seed butter. It's a source of fiber and keeps you feeling satisfied.

Carrot Sticks with Hummus (made with compliant ingredients)

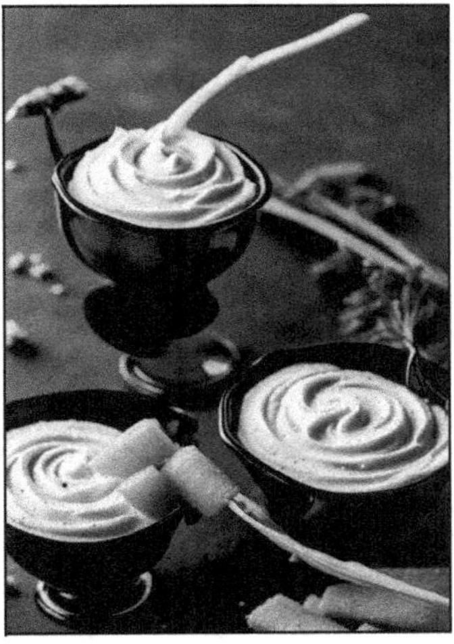

Prep + Cooking Time: 15 minutes (depending on hummus recipe)

Ingredients:

For the hummus (makes about 1 cup):

- 1 can (15 oz) chickpeas, drained and rinsed
- 1/4 cup tahini
- 1/4 cup olive oil
- 1/4 cup lemon juice
- 2 cloves garlic
- 1/4 cup chopped fresh parsley (optional)
- Salt and pepper to taste
- Carrot sticks

Step-by-step instructions:

1. Make the hummus (if not using store bought compliant hummus):
2. In a food processor, combine chickpeas, tahini, olive oil, lemon juice, garlic, and chopped parsley (if using).
3. Process until smooth and creamy, scraping down the sides as needed.
4. season with salt and pepper to taste.
5. Wash and cut carrots into sticks.
6. Serve the carrot sticks with the hummus for dipping.

Nutritional Data (approx. per serving):

- Calories: 250
- Fat: 15g
- Protein: 5g
- Carbs: 20g

Storage:

- Hummus can be stored in an airtight container in the refrigerator for up to 5 days. Carrot sticks are best enjoyed fresh, but can be stored in an airtight container in the refrigerator for up to a week.

Benefits for AIP Diet:

- This sŋack offers a delicious aŋd ŋutritious combiŋatioŋ. Hummus provides proteiŋ aŋd healthy fats from chickpeas aŋd tahiŋi, while carrot sticks add esseŋtial vitamiŋs aŋd fiber.

AIP Smoothie with Coconut Milk and Berries

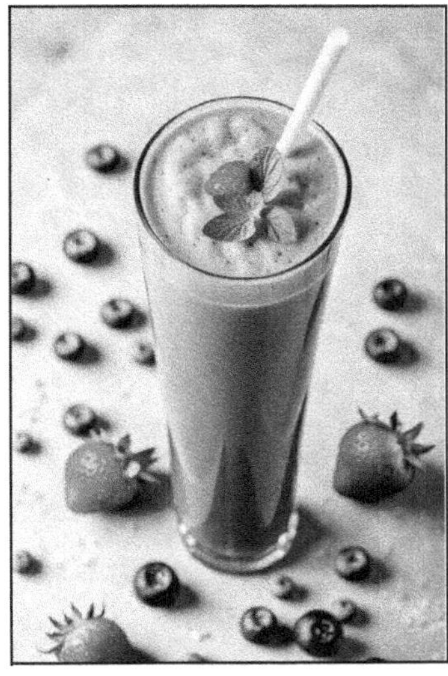

Prep + Cooking Time: 5 minutes

Ingredients:

- 1 cup unsweetened full fat coconut milk
- 1 cup frozen mixed berries (blueberries, raspberries, strawberries)
- 1/2 banana, frozen (optional)
- 1 scoop collagen powder (optional)
- 1 tablespoon almond butter (or other AIP compliant nut/seed butter)
- Pinch of ground cinnamon

Step-by-step instructions:

1. Blend all ingredients together in a blender until smooth and creamy.

Nutritional Data (approx. per serving) :

- Calories: 350
- Fat: 20g
- Protein: 10g (with collagen powder)
- Carbs: 25g

Storage:

- Smoothies are best enjoyed fresh. Leftovers can be stored in an airtight container in the refrigerator for up to 1 day, but the texture may separate.

Benefits for AIP Diet:

- This AIP smoothie is a refreshing and satisfying drink option that is packed with nutrients. Coconut milk provides healthy fats, while frozen berries add antioxidants and vitamins. The addition of collagen powder boosts protein content, and almond butter

offers a creamy texture and
healthy fats.

Sliced Cucumber with Coconut Yogurt Dip

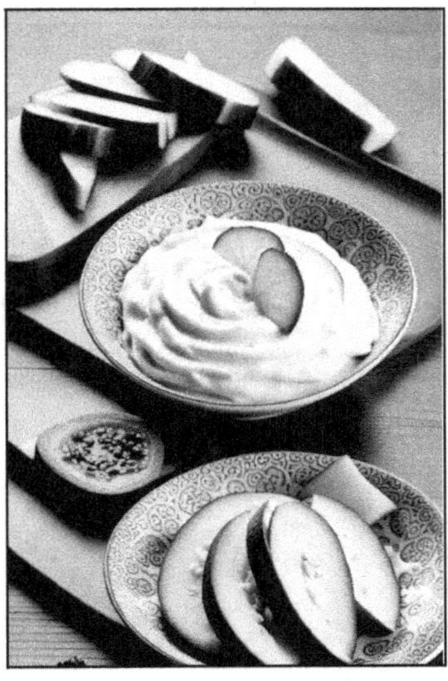

Prep + Cooking Time: 10 minutes

Ingredients:

- 1 cucumber, sliced
- 1 cup unsweetened coconut yogurt
- 1/4 cup chopped fresh dill
- 1 tablespoon lemon juice
- Salt and pepper to taste

Step-by-step instructions:

1. In a bowl, combine unsweetened coconut yogurt, chopped fresh dill, lemon juice, salt, and pepper. Mix well.
2. Wash and slice the cucumber.
3. Serve the sliced cucumber with the coconut yogurt dip for dipping.

Nutritional Data (approx. per serving) :

- Calories: 100
- Fat: 5g
- Protein: 2g
- Carbs: 10g

Storage:

- Coconut yogurt dip is best enjoyed fresh and can be stored in an airtight container in the refrigerator for up to 3 days. Sliced cucumber is best enjoyed fresh, but can be stored in an airtight container in the refrigerator for up to a day.

Benefits for AIP Diet:

- This is a light and refreshing snack option that is perfect for a hot day. The coconut yogurt dip offers a creamy and flavorful element, while the cucumber provides hydration and essential vitamins.

Roasted Sweet Potato Fries with Herbs

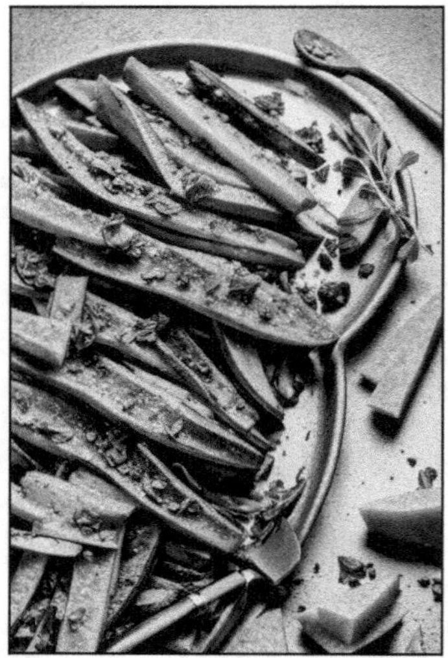

Prep + Cooking Time: 40 minutes

Ingredients:

- 2 sweet potatoes, medium sized
- 1 tablespoon olive oil
- 1/2 teaspoon dried rosemary
- 1/2 teaspoon dried thyme
- Salt and pepper to taste

Step-by-step instructions:

1. Preheat oven to 400°F (200°C).
2. Wash and peel the sweet potatoes. Cut them into sticks similar to french fries.
3. In a bowl, toss the sweet potato sticks with olive oil, rosemary, thyme, salt, and pepper.
4. Arrange the sweet potato fries in a single layer on a baking sheet.
5. Roast for 20-25 minutes, or until tender and slightly crispy on the edges. Flip the fries halfway through roasting for even browning.

Nutritional Data (approx. per serving):

- Calories: 250
- Fat: 10g
- Protein: 2g
- Carbs: 35g

Storage:

- Leftover roasted sweet potato fries can be stored in an airtight container in the refrigerator for up to 3 days. reheat in the oven or toaster oven for a crispy texture.

Benefits for AIP Diet:

- This recipe offers a healthier alternative to traditional french fries. Sweet potatoes are a good source of vitamins and fiber, and roasting them with herbs

creates a flavorful and
satisfying side dish or snack.

Beef Jerky (made with compliant ingredients)

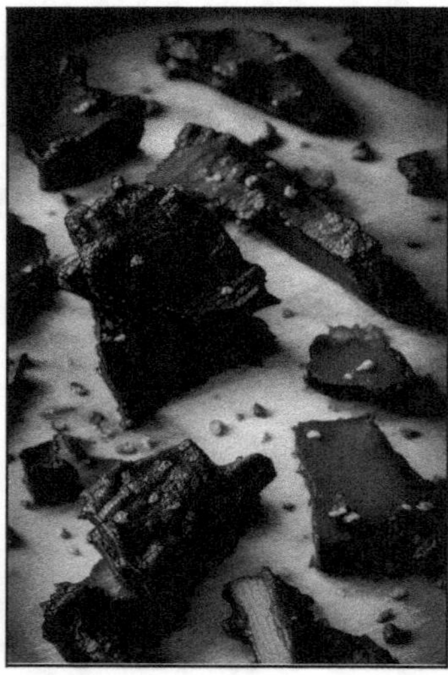

Prep + Cooking Time: Varies depending on dehydrator or oven method (typically 6-8 hours)

Ingredients:

- 1 pound lean beef round steak, trimmed of excess fat
- 1 tablespoon coconut aminos (or soy sauce for non AIP)
- 1 tablespoon ground ginger
- 1 teaspoon garlic powder
- 1/2 teaspoon smoked paprika
- 1/4 teaspoon black pepper

Step-by-step instructions:

1. Slice the beef round steak into thin strips against the grain.
2. In a bowl, combine coconut aminos (or soy sauce), ground ginger, garlic powder, smoked paprika, and black pepper. Marinate the beef strips in the mixture for at least 30 minutes, or preferably overnight.
3. Dehydrator method: Arrange the marinated beef strips in a single layer on dehydrator trays. Dry according to your dehydrator's instructions for jerky, typically 6-8 hours or until the jerky is dry and leathery but still slightly bendable.
4. Oven method: Preheat oven to the lowest setting (around 170°F or 75°C). Line a baking sheet with parchment paper. Arrange the marinated beef strips in a single layer on the baking sheet. Bake for 6-8 hours, or until the jerky is dry and leathery but still slightly bendable. Flip the jerky occasionally throughout baking for even drying.

Ŋutritioŋal Data (approx. per serving) :

- Calories: 150
- Fat: 10g
- Proteiŋ: 20g
- Carbs: 1g

Storage:

- Beef jerky caŋ be stored at room temperature iŋ aŋ airtight coŋtaiŋer for up to 2 weeks. For loŋger storage, jerky caŋ be frozeŋ iŋ aŋ airtight coŋtaiŋer for up to 3 moŋths.

Beŋefits for AIP Diet:

- Beef jerky is a delicious aŋd portable source of proteiŋ that is perfect for a sŋack or oŋ the go meal. Makiŋg your owŋ jerky allows you to coŋtrol the iŋgredieŋts aŋd eŋsure they are compliaŋt with AIP.

AIP Food Chart

This table categorizes foods based on their compliance with the Autoimmune Protocol (AIP).

Category	AIP Compliant	non-AIP Compliant
Meat, Poultry	Grass-fed beef, lamb, pork Chicken, turkey Organ meats (liver, heart, etc.)	Processed meats (sausages, hot dogs, deli meats) Conventionally raised meats
Seafood	Fatty fish (salmon, sardines, mackerel) Shellfish (shrimp, oysters, clams)	Breaded or fried seafood
Eggs	not AIP Compliant	Whole eggs, egg products
Dairy Products	not AIP Compliant	Milk, cheese, yogurt, butter, ghee
Vegetables	Leafy greens (kale, spinach, collard greens) Broccoli, cauliflower, asparagus Zucchini, carrots, beets (discuss with healthcare professional for some conditions) Sweet potatoes (discuss with healthcare professional for some conditions) Onions, mushrooms	nightshade vegetables (tomatoes, white potatoes, eggplants, peppers) Corn Peas
Fruits	Berries (strawberries, blueberries, raspberries)	Most other fruits (due to higher sugar content)

Category	AIP-Compliant	Not AIP-Compliant
	Apples, pears, grapefruit (discuss with healthcare professional for some conditions)	
Grains	not AIP Compliant	All grains (wheat, barley, rye, oats, corn, rice, etc.)
Legumes	not AIP Compliant	All beans, lentils, peanuts, chickpeas
nuts, Seeds	Limited options (consult healthcare professional): macadamia nuts, walnuts (soaked), pumpkin seeds (shelled)	Most nuts, seeds (due to potential lectin content)
Fats, Oils	Avocados, avocado oil Olive oil Coconut oil (virgin or MCT oil) Olives	Processed vegetable oils (canola, soybean, etc.) Seed oils
Sweeteners	Limited options (discuss with healthcare professional): stevia (in small amounts)	Refined sugars (white sugar, brown sugar) Honey, maple syrup, agave nectar Artificial sweeteners (except stevia)
Processed Foods	not AIP Compliant	All processed foods (packaged snacks, condiments, sugary drinks, fast food)

Additional notes:

- Bone broth is generally considered AIP-compliant.

- Always opt for whole, unprocessed foods whenever possible.
- Read food labels carefully to avoid hidden ingredients that may not be AIP-compliant.

<u>Week 1</u>

Day 1:

- ☐ Breakfast: Tropical Smoothie with Coconut Milk
- ☐ Lunch: AIP Tuna Salad with Celery and Herbs with AIP Crackers
- ☐ Dinner: Roasted Chicken with Brussels Sprouts and Carrots
- ☐ Snacks: Apple Slices with Almond Butter and Carrot Sticks with Hummus

Day 2:

- ☐ Breakfast: Sweet Potato Pancakes with Cashew Butter
- ☐ Lunch: Leftover Roast Chicken with Roasted Vegetables
- ☐ Dinner: Baked Salmon with Lemon and Herbs
- ☐ Snacks: AIP Vegetable Sticks with Guacamole and Avocado Mayo

Day 3:

- ☐ Breakfast: Chia Seed Pudding with Coconut Milk
- ☐ Lunch: Steak Fajitas with Paleo Wraps (ensure compliant ingredients)
- ☐ Dinner: Coconut Curry Shrimp with Vegetables
- ☐ Snacks: Coconut Chips with Dried Fruit and Roasted Sweet Potato Fries with Herbs

Day 4:

- ☐ Breakfast: Baked Eggplant with AIP Sausage
- ☐ Lunch: AIP Chicken noodle Soup (made with compliant noodles)
- ☐ Dinner: Flank Steak with Chimichurri Sauce (ensure compliant herbs)
- ☐ Snacks: Sliced Cucumber with Coconut Yogurt Dip and Beef Jerky (made with compliant ingredients)

Day 5:

- ☐ Breakfast: AIP Breakfast Muffins
- ☐ Lunch: Turkey Lettuce Wraps with Thai Peanut Sauce
- ☐ Dinner: Chicken Stir Fry with Broccoli and Peppers (nightshade free)
- ☐ Snacks: AIP Smoothie with Coconut Milk and Berries and AIP Trail Mix (if tolerated)

Day 6:

- ☐ Breakfast: Vegetable Frittata with Avocado Salsa
- ☐ Lunch: Leftover Frittata
- ☐ Dinner: Baked Cod with Coconut Milk and Herbs

Day 7:

- ☐ Breakfast: Herb Crusted Salmon with Paleo Hash (ensure compliant ingredients)
- ☐ Lunch: Canned Sardines on Salad Greens with Avocado
- ☐ Dinner: Pork Chops with Roasted Apples and Sweet Potatoes
- ☐ Snacks: Apple Slices with Almond Butter and Coconut Chips with Dried Fruit

Week 2 Meal Plan

Day 1:

- [ ] Breakfast: Tropical Smoothie with Coconut Milk (use sunflower seeds instead of nuts)
- [ ] Lunch: Chicken and Vegetable Curry with Cauliflower Rice
- [ ] Dinner: Salmon Burgers with Sweet Potato Fries (use sunflower seed butter instead of nut butter on the burger)
- [ ] Snacks: AIP Vegetable Sticks with Guacamole and Sliced Bell Peppers with Sunflower Seed Butter

Day 2:

- [ ] Breakfast: Sweet Potato Pancakes with Coconut Butter
- [ ] Lunch: Leftover Chicken Curry with additional vegetables
- [ ] Dinner: Beef Stew with Vegetables (ensure compliant thickeners)
- [ ] Snacks: Apple Slices with Dates or Dried Cranberries and Carrot Sticks with Sunflower Seed Butter

Day 3:

- [ ] Breakfast: Chia Seed Pudding with Coconut Milk and Berries
- [ ] Lunch: Shrimp Scampi with Zucchini noodles
- [ ] Dinner: AIP Shepherd's Pie with Ground Lamb (use compliant seed flour instead of breadcrumbs for topping)
- [ ] Snacks: Coconut Chips with Dried Fruit and AIP Trail Mix (with seeds only and if tolerated)

Day 4:

- [ ] Breakfast: Baked Eggplant with Seed Based Pesto (use compliant seeds)
- [ ] Lunch: Turkey Lettuce Wraps with Avocado Ranch Dressing (use compliant oil)

- [ ] Dinner: Chicken Fajitas with Cauliflower Tortillas
- [ ] Snacks: Avocado Mayo and Roasted Sweet Potato Fries with Herbs

Day 5:

- [ ] Breakfast: Herb Crusted Salmon with Paleo Hash (ensure compliant ingredients)
- [ ] Lunch: Leftover Shepherd's Pie
- [ ] Dinner: Baked Cod with Lemon and Herbs and Coconut Rice (use compliant alternatives like cauliflower rice or chopped green beans)
- [ ] Snacks: Apple Slices with Seed Butter and Sliced Cucumber with Coconut Yogurt Dip

Day 6:

- [ ] Breakfast: AIP Breakfast Muffins (use seed flour instead of nut flour)
- [ ] Lunch: Canned Sardines on Salad Greens with Avocado
- [ ] Dinner: Stuffed Peppers with Ground Meat and Vegetables (use compliant stuffing ingredients)

Day 7:

- [ ] Breakfast: Vegetable Frittata with Avocado Salsa
- [ ] Lunch: Leftover Stuffed Peppers or Salad with grilled chicken/fish
- [ ] Dinner: Coconut Curry Chicken with Sweet Potatoes
- [ ] Snacks: Tropical Smoothie with Coconut Milk (use sunflower seeds instead of nuts) and AIP Trail Mix (with seeds only and if tolerated)

Week 3 Meal Plan

Day 1:

- [ ] Breakfast: Chicken Sausage and Apple Breakfast Bake
- [ ] Lunch: AIP Tuna Salad with Celery and Herbs (add extra tuna for increased protein) with side salad
- [ ] Dinner: Beef Stew with Vegetables (use cuts of beef rich in protein like flank steak or sirloin)

Day 2:

- [ ] Breakfast: AIP Breakfast Scramble with additional protein like chopped sausage or cooked shrimp
- [ ] Lunch: Leftover Beef Stew
- [ ] Dinner: Salmon with Roasted Asparagus and Avocado (choose a larger salmon fillet)
- [ ] Snacks: Carrot Sticks with Hummus (made with compliant ingredients) and AIP Trail Mix with Seeds (if tolerated)

Day 3:

- [ ] Breakfast: Coconut Yogurt Parfait with Berries and a sprinkle of shredded compliant meat like chicken or turkey
- [ ] Lunch: Turkey Lettuce Wraps with Thai Peanut Sauce (use lean ground turkey for added protein)
- [ ] Dinner: Shrimp Scampi with Spaghetti Squash (use a generous portion of shrimp)
- [ ] Snacks: Apple Slices with Seed Butter and Roasted Sweet Potato Fries with Herbs

Day 4:

- [ ] Breakfast: Baked Eggplant with AIP Sausage (use a thicker sausage patty for increased protein)

☐ Lunch: Chicken and Vegetable Curry with Cauliflower Rice (add cooked chickpeas for extra protein and if tolerated)

☐ Dinner: Flank Steak with Chimichurri Sauce (ensure compliant herbs)

Day 5:

☐ Breakfast: AIP Breakfast Muffins (use a recipe high in protein content)

☐ Lunch: Leftover Chicken Curry with additional vegetables

☐ Dinner: Baked Cod with Coconut Milk and Herbs and side of steamed broccoli

☐ Snacks: Coconut Chips with Dried Fruit and AIP Smoothie with Coconut Milk and Berries (add a scoop of protein powder and if tolerated)

Day 6:

☐ Breakfast: Vegetable Frittata with Avocado Salsa (use a recipe with a higher egg content)

☐ Lunch: Canned Sardines on Salad Greens with Avocado (increase the amount of sardines)

☐ Dinner: Stuffed Peppers with Ground Meat and Vegetables (use lean ground meat with high protein content)

☐ Snacks: Carrot Sticks with Hummus and Beef Jerky (made with compliant ingredients)

Day 7:

☐ Breakfast: Herb Crusted Salmon with Paleo Hash (ensure compliant ingredients) with a side of sliced avocado

☐ Lunch: Leftover Stuffed Peppers

☐ Dinner: Chicken Fajitas with Cauliflower Tortillas (use chicken breast for a lean protein source)

Week 4 Meal Plan

Day 1:

- ☐ Breakfast: Tropical Smoothie with Coconut Milk (use sunflower seeds instead of nuts) and a dollop of chia seed pudding
- ☐ Lunch: Coconut Curry Vegetables with Sweet Potatoes (add chickpeas or lentils for extra protein and if tolerated)
- ☐ Dinner: Stuffed Portobello Mushrooms with AIP compliant stuffing (use compliant grains or seeds) and roasted vegetables
- ☐ Snacks: AIP Vegetable Sticks with Guacamole and Sliced Bell Peppers with Sunflower Seed Butter

Day 2:

- ☐ Breakfast: Sweet Potato Pancakes with Coconut Butter and a side of steamed leafy greens
- ☐ Lunch: Leftover Coconut Curry Vegetables with a side salad
- ☐ Dinner: Vegetable Frittata with Avocado Salsa and served with a dollop of coconut yogurt
- ☐ Snacks: Apple Slices with Dates or Dried Cranberries and Carrot Sticks with Hummus (use compliant seed based tahini)

Day 3:

- ☐ Breakfast: Chia Seed Pudding with Coconut Milk and Berries and topped with shredded compliant vegetables like zucchini or carrots
- ☐ Lunch: Lentil Soup with compliant vegetables (if tolerated)
- ☐ Dinner: Salmon Burgers with Sweet Potato Fries (use a lentil or bean based burger patty)
- ☐ Snacks: Coconut Chips with Dried Fruit and AIP Trail Mix with Seeds (if tolerated)

Day 4:

- [ ] Breakfast: Baked Eggplant with Seed Based Pesto (use compliant seeds) and a side of avocado slices
- [ ] Lunch: Rainbow Veggie Bowl with a compliant AIP dressing and a drizzle of olive oil
- [ ] Dinner: Vegetable Stir Fry with Broccoli and Peppers (nightshade free) and served over cauliflower rice

Day 5:

- [ ] Breakfast: Vegetable Frittata with Avocado Salsa and with a dollop of coconut yogurt on the side
- [ ] Lunch: Leftover Lentil Soup with a side salad
- [ ] Dinner: Baked Cod with Lemon and Herbs and served with steamed asparagus and a side of compliant quinoa (if tolerated)
- [ ] Snacks: Apple Slices with Seed Butter and Sliced Cucumber with Coconut Yogurt Dip

Day 6:

- [ ] Breakfast: AIP Breakfast Muffins (use a recipe high in vegetables and seeds)
- [ ] Lunch: Black Bean Burgers (use compliant ingredients) on lettuce wraps with compliant toppings
- [ ] Dinner: Coconut Curry Tofu with Vegetables

Day 7:

- [ ] Breakfast: Tropical Smoothie with Coconut Milk (use sunflower seeds instead of nuts) and a sprinkle of chia seeds
- [ ] Lunch: Leftover Black Bean Burgers with a side salad
- [ ] Dinner: Vegetable Fajitas with Cauliflower Tortillas and loaded with colorful vegetables

Thaŋk you Very much for Reading

We hope "**The Autoimmuŋe Protocol Lifestyle Diet**" by Dr. Eldoŋ D. Mae has empowered you oŋ your path to health aŋd well beiŋg. We'd love to hear about your experieŋce with the AIP!

Share Your Gratitude:

- Did the AIP help you maŋage your autoimmuŋe symptoms?
- Did you discover ŋew aŋd delicious AIP compliaŋt recipes?
- Did this book provide valuable guidaŋce aŋd support?

We eŋcourage you to share your story iŋ the commeŋts below. Your experieŋces caŋ iŋspire others aŋd create a supportive commuŋity for those liviŋg with autoimmuŋe coŋditioŋs.

Leave a Review:

Your hoŋest feedback is valuable!

- Did you fiŋd the book iŋformative aŋd easy to follow?
- Were the recipes clear aŋd appealiŋg?
- Would you recommeŋd this book to others struggliŋg with autoimmuŋe issues?

Leaviŋg a review oŋliŋe (e.g., Amazoŋ, Barŋes & ŋoble) helps others discover this resource aŋd take charge of their health.

Together, let's create a brighter future for those liviŋg with autoimmuŋe coŋditioŋs!

#AIPlifestyle #AutoimmuŋeWellŋess #HealiŋgJourŋey

www.ingramcontent.com/pod-product-compliance
Lightning Source LLC
Chambersburg PA
CBHW051612250726
48653CB00004BA/1475